Praise for *Creating*

"This book should be read by every woman planning to give birth."
—Ina May Gaskin, author of *Ina May's Guide to Childbirth* and *Spiritual Midwifery*

"It is critical for every mother to be an active and vocal partner with her care provider throughout her pregnancy and childbirth, to ensure a safe and good experience. Dr. Wagner's book offers valuable insights into the many decisions pregnant women face."
—Tonya Jamois, President, International Cesarean Awareness Network

"This must-read book will alleviate your fear of birth and help guide you to the best birth possible. It will put you in control and bring you the miracle that is awaiting you and your baby."
—Jan Tritten, leading U.S. midwife and director of Midwifery Today

"This is the guide you need to planning the birth you want, the birth you and your baby deserve—a loving, empowering, healthy, joyous birth."
—Barbara Katz Rothman, Professor of Sociology, City University of New York

continued . . .

"Here is a clear and complete explanation of 'woman-centered childbirth,' including practical, realistic advice and step-by-step guidance for planning a safe and empowering birth, as *you* define it."

—Penny Simkin, author of *The Birth Partner: Everything You Need to Know to Help a Woman Through Childbirth*

"*Creating Your Birth Plan* is fantastic. As a childbirth educator for twenty years, I find it holds exactly the right information that women and their partners need to navigate the maze of technology and options that are available as they develop their birth preferences. I plan to make this wonderful book required reading for my classes, and I hope every pregnant woman will choose to read it."

—Debra Pascali-Bonaro, certified childbirth educator, leading trainer of childbirth educators and doulas

"Just as professionals use textbooks to guide their care, mothers should have textbooks to guide the way they want their care to be managed! This is one such textbook. It is imperative that healthcare providers make books like this available to the most important member of the healthcare team . . . the mother."

—Juliana van Olphen Fehr, CNM, PhD, FACNM, Coordinator, Nurse-Midwifery, Shenandoah University

Creating Your
Birth Plan

*The Definitive Guide
to a Safe and Empowering Birth*

Marsden Wagner, M.D., M.S.
with Stephanie Gunning

A Perigee Book

THE BERKLEY PUBLISHING GROUP
Published by the Penguin Group
Penguin Group (USA) Inc.
375 Hudson Street, New York, New York 10014, USA
Penguin Group (Canada), 90 Eglinton Avenue East, Suite 700, Toronto, Ontario M4P 2Y3, Canada
(a division of Pearson Penguin Canada Inc.)
Penguin Books Ltd., 80 Strand, London WC2R 0RL, England
Penguin Group Ireland, 25 St. Stephen's Green, Dublin 2, Ireland (a division of Penguin Books Ltd.)
Penguin Group (Australia), 250 Camberwell Road, Camberwell, Victoria 3124, Australia
(a division of Pearson Australia Group Pty. Ltd.)
Penguin Books India Pvt. Ltd., 11 Community Centre, Panchsheel Park, New Delhi—110 017, India
Penguin Group (NZ), Cnr. Airborne and Rosedale Roads, Albany, Auckland 1310, New Zealand
(a division of Pearson New Zealand Ltd.)
Penguin Books (South Africa) (Pty.) Ltd., 24 Sturdee Avenue, Rosebank, Johannesburg 2196, South Africa

Penguin Books Ltd., Registered Offices: 80 Strand, London WC2R 0RL, England

While the author has made every effort to provide accurate telephone numbers and Internet addresses at the time of publication, neither the publisher nor the author assumes any responsibility for errors, or for changes that occur after publication. Further, publisher does not have any control over and does not assume any responsibility for author or third-party websites or their content.

First edition: June 2006

Library of Congress Cataloging-in-Publication Data

Wagner, Marsden, 1930–
  Creating your birth plan : the definitive guide to a safe and empowering birth / Marsden Wagner with Stephanie Gunning.
      p.   cm.
  Includes bibliographical references and index.
  ISBN 0-399-53257-9
  1. Birth plans.   2. Childbirth.   3. Labor (Obstetrics)—Popular works.   I. Gunning, Stephanie, 1962–   II. Title.
    RG652.W26   2006
    618.4—dc22   2006044773

PRINTED IN THE UNITED STATES OF AMERICA

10 9 8 7 6 5 4 3 2 1

PUBLISHER'S NOTE: The information contained in this book is not a substitute for professional medical advice. While the advice and information in this book are believed to be true and accurate at the date of going to press, neither the author nor the publisher can accept any legal responsibility for any errors or omissions that may be made. The publisher makes no warranty, express or implied, with respect to the material contained herein. Readers should consult their physician or midwife before acting on any of the information contained in this volume.

To my family
You give me courage and joy,
and you mean everything to me

Acknowledgments

My gratitude goes to Stephanie Gunning, the perfect coauthor; Stephany Evans, the agent who is always there; and Meg Leder, so helpful with the book's editing. For exceptional generosity in sharing their professional perspectives and personal accounts of childbirth, many sincere thanks are also due to Lowell Levin, Ina May Gaskin, Leslie Whitcomb, Deborah Badran, Kelly Townsend, Dana Parness, Heidi Rinehart, Maddy Oden, Tanja Johnson, Natalie Laughlin, Sandy Grason, Patricia Stephenson, Peggy Vincent, Steve Schuetze, Mark Bower, Diana and Marco North, Jan Tritten, Robbie Davis-Floyd, Juliana Fehr, Sheryl Rivett, Henci Goer, Murray Enkin, Chris Kjellsen, Kathleen Steinberg, Susan Hodges, Barbara Katz Rothman, Saraswathi Vedam, Caroline Rafferty, Katherine Prown, Tonya Jamois, Steve Cochran, everyone in the Coalition for Improvement of Maternity Services, Baby-Friendly USA, Childbirth Connection, and the Metropolitan Doula Group of New York.

Contents

Creating Your

Birth Plan

Introduction

Creating Your Birth Plan

Creating Your Birth Plan: The Definitive Guide to a Safe and Empowering Birth is a book about using a birth plan in working toward a woman-centered childbirth. A birth plan is an approach to labor, rather than a term for a specific kind of outcome. Many aspects of labor are impossible to plan for, such as the speed of dilation and the strength of your next contraction. This book is designed to support you in achieving your goals for an ideal childbirth process.

If you are pregnant or you are planning to become pregnant, you have more options and issues to consider today than at any other time in history. As perhaps the most important set of healthcare decisions you will ever make, you need and deserve to have unbiased facts—both the pros and the cons—about the different types of maternity care available to you. You are entitled to excellent labor support and fully informed consent. No matter how the course of labor unfolds, you, as the pregnant woman at the center of it all, have ultimate responsibility for creating an experience for yourself that is as safe, stress free, and satisfying as possible. You are entitled to plan and then enjoy the birth experience of your dreams, as much as the mysteries of nature allow.

Giving birth is an exciting, awe-inspiring, and life-altering event. Long before becoming a mother, a pregnant woman already feels responsible for the baby she is carrying. For months, she anticipates change and ponders its meaning. Simultaneously, her body goes through a metamorphosis to prepare her for labor. At the end of pregnancy, what would have been inconceivable at another time is now actually possible—an eight-pound (or so) human being emerging into the world through her vagina. Yet childbirth is rarely unremarkable or ordinary. There simply are too many factors involved.

It doesn't matter how many children you have carried, no one can predict exactly what the labor experience will be like for you—long or brief, painful, euphoric, difficult or easy—or if any complications will arise in the process. Childbirth requires your physical, mental, and emotional stamina. While it brings up feelings of joy, hope, and love, it can also stir up numerous fears: of the unknown, of your ability (or lack of ability), of trauma and pain, and about safety for your child and you. During childbirth, you may feel defenseless and overwhelmed. But there is a way to make this significant and emotionally supercharged event more tranquil and easier to handle. And your ability to relax and trust those around you is a key factor in safer and more pleasurable labor.

Creating Your Birth Plan will help you to create a personalized birth plan, a signed document that clearly indicates to your professional caregivers your preferences and decisions about the assistance you will receive. It can help you inform them of your standards for decision-making in case of emergency. In the current climate of care, a birth plan may be the most effective tool you can have to exercise a degree of control and trust during your childbirth. (Of course, many aspects of childbirth are not under anyone's control!) Because it is an educational process, designing a birth plan prepares you for childbirth. It teaches you about your options. It helps you evaluate the risks and benefits of various interventions. It assuages unnecessary fears. A birth plan empowers you to make good choices at every step of the way. Creating a personalized birth plan is not an adversarial process; however, if you find yourself in disagreement with your caregivers, the birth plan also can give you a measure of legal leverage. It gives you a legitimate means to express your voice during an exciting but vulnerable passage in your life.

Why This Book Is Needed
—⟋

More than four million American women give birth each year, with more than 95 percent of them in hospitals. They choose hospitals for a variety of reasons having to do with the incorrect idea that hospitals can provide the safest births. Although women sometimes choose to labor in hospitals because they have no access to a home-birth midwife, or because an insurance company mandates the decision, often it's because they believe that a doctor can guarantee their safety in case of an emergency. While midwives oversee some hospital births, obstetricians and labor-and-delivery nurses manage the majority. Another reason women choose hospitals is to have access to strong pain medication—epidurals.

As a result of our reliance on hospitals and doctors, birth in America has come to be perceived as a medical event rather than a natural one—we literally view it through the eyes of doctors. We spend twice as much as any other country in the world per birth, because medical technology and drugs are highly esteemed and widely available, and we want to purchase the best care. Even in normal pregnancies, our rate for interventions, like electronic fetal monitoring, labor induction and augmentation, and cesarean section, is skyrocketing. Nonetheless, many other countries get better results than we do using less technology and fewer medications.[1] What are the pregnant women and the maternity caregivers in those countries doing or not doing that would benefit you?

Creating Your Birth Plan will explore the standards of care in hospitals, out-of-hospital birth centers, and at-home births. According to scientific evidence, do hospitals and doctors adhere to the best and safest practices? Do midwives adhere to the best and safest practices? Under what types of emergency conditions is it important to be under the care of an obstetrician? What factors are valuable for you to take into consideration before giving birth in a hospital, in an independent birth center, or at home? What would a truly natural birth, one without any interventions and medications, be like?

As an expectant mother you need to be an active participant in your own care. You need to know how to recognize excellent professional caregivers as well as how to protect yourself from the less-scrupulous type of practitioners who allow fear of litigation to influence their decision-making about childbirth and outweigh research studies.

As a physician and scientist, and a former director of Women's and Children's Health at the World Health Organization (WHO), I headed a team for fifteen years that gathered scientific data on different forms of maternity care throughout the world's industrialized nations. We investigated everything from laboring postures and whether or not a woman should eat, drink, and move around, to the efficacy of electronic fetal monitoring, ultrasound, intravenous drips, anesthesia, episiotomies, forceps and vacuum extraction, and cesarean section. *Creating Your Birth Plan* incorporates those findings.

In America today, there is often profound misunderstanding and mistrust of the midwifery model of care that other highly industrialized countries worldwide embrace and find essential for the management of normal, healthy labor. Statistics have shown that home birth and hospital birth managed by midwives tend to be safest for women and their babies, as well as most fulfilling. Hopefully this book can help you understand midwives, so that you can carefully evaluate the services they provide based on facts, not myths.

Producing a healthy baby is a major goal of birth. But a successful birth outcome involves so much more than mere survival. We should not disregard the human impact of childbirth. Positive laboring experiences set women up to become good mothers and more confident people. Some people climb mountains or run marathons to find out what they are capable of. Giving birth presents a comparable opportunity for the woman who decides to become a mother. It can reveal her to herself and transform her self-image.

Considering everything we know about birth and its significance, how can you and your loved ones ensure that the birth of your child is as safe and as satisfying as possible? With a personalized birth plan, no matter where you choose to labor and whom you select to be your primary birth attendant, you can.

How to Use This Book

When we discuss the creation of a birth plan, what we're really discussing is a multifaceted process. First, you need information about everything that could happen. Second, you need information about different ways to handle what happens. Third, you need to make decisions about your preferences in case things happen. And finally, you need to communicate or express those preferences.

To get you started on your information-gathering process, *Creating Your Birth Plan* shares information I've gathered from interviews with forward-thinking obstetricians, midwives, doulas, and public health experts, as well as actual birth stories, in addition to my own firsthand experiences and knowledge. The text also incorporates the latest scientific research drawn from leading sources in the field of maternity care, such as the Cochrane Library and the World Health Organization, as well as statistics drawn from valid international scientific studies conducted in countries that include the United Kingdom, Brazil, Germany, New Zealand, and Japan, and by organizations in the United States such as the National Association of Childbearing Centers and Childbirth Connection (formerly the Maternity Center Association). Two attorneys specializing in medical malpractice have been consulted on legal matters.

This book is organized so you can understand the different factors that directly influence the hands-on care that pregnant women, women in labor, and newborn babies receive. Serious issues are occasionally raised about the current system of childbirth. You'll find practical information on how you and your family can protect yourselves and ensure that you get the best possible care and have a positive birthing experience.

Creating Your Birth Plan will help you evaluate the following issues:

- Where do you want to give birth—in a hospital, an out-of-hospital birthing center, or at home—and what typically takes place in these environments?

- What type of clinical caregiver would you prefer to assist you during labor—a doctor or a midwife—and how do their training and approaches differ?

- How can you evaluate and communicate with the caregiver you've selected?

- Who should be your advocate to ensure that your caregivers honor your wishes and decisions—for example, a spouse or life partner, a family member, and/or a doula?

- Who would you like to offer you emotional support?

- What are the natural stages of labor in a problem-free birth?

- What are the possible complications you could face?

- What kinds of medical or surgical interventions could you need or choose? And what are their potential risks and benefits?

- Are there natural alternatives to drugs, technology, and surgery?

- What has science shown to be the most helpful and safest laboring practices?

- What are your dreams, expectations, and feelings about labor?

Every chapter in *Creating Your Birth Plan* is organized around the theme of designing and implementing a birth plan. The goal is first to inform you, and then to arm you with a series of valuable questions to ask your caregiver if relevant matters arise. Understanding the realities of birth—and your human and legal rights as the central figure in the birth experience—will help you to allay many of your fears. It will also help safeguard you and your unborn baby against unwarranted medical procedures, so that you and your baby have as safe a birth as possible.

Chapter 1 introduces the gold standard of maternity care and addresses matters relating to why birth should be woman centered. Chapter 2 explains the stages of normal, uncomplicated labor that the great majority of healthy women may anticipate. Reading chapter 3, you'll contemplate various planned birth locations where you could enjoy a normal birth: your home, different types of birth centers, and a hospital. In chapter 4, you'll weigh the pros and cons of doctors and midwives in attending normal births. The conjoined decisions of location and caregiver will help lay the foundation of your plan.

Chapters 5 through 8 examine possible complications and possible interventions using drugs and surgery that you may experience. Can you avoid such procedures? What alternatives are available to you to handle each problem? Here you'll learn the answers.

In chapters 9 through 12, you'll learn about support systems, high-risk and low-risk conditions (both the physical and emotional), baby-friendly care, and your postpartum recovery period.

Finally, you'll put all your knowledge to work in the actual plan you'll draft when reading chapter 13. Organized in the form of a review from earlier chapters, a great benefit of putting your ideas on paper is having the opportunity to visualize the overall arc of the labor and birth you're going to undergo, along with being given ideas about how to express your wishes and protect your rights.

Women and their partners desire exhilarating and transformational childbirth experiences, yet often sacrifice these *needlessly* for the sake of false security. As a doctor and a specialist in maternity care, I would like to help guide you through the maze of maternity-care decisions you make now and in the future. With this book, my intention is to support you to have both safety and the meaningful, even sacred childbirth you are seeking. Whatever you ultimately choose, I hope it exceeds your expectations.

One

Principles of Woman-Centered Care

The first time I was present at a natural, unmedicated birth a transformation took place near the end of the woman's labor. Her face began to glow and she shouted her feelings of determination to everyone within earshot. She was going to do this! The moment she pushed the baby out of her body, she triumphantly yelled, "I did it!" Then she leaned over, took her newborn infant in her arms, and looked around the room proudly, wearing an angelic expression that would have put Michelangelo to shame. It was awe inspiring. Every woman should feel as much pride and euphoria at her labor's end.

As for me, at that moment my understanding of childbirth would never be the same. Even with all my experience as a physician, it was surprising for me to see a woman give birth in her full power and autonomy: making strange sounds, moving however she wanted to make herself comfortable, and clearly demanding her needs be met—and having her birth attendants support all her choices. It was unlike most hospital births. I had been trained to take charge of birth and use my medical skills to make sure that women in labor wouldn't be harmed, to manage the risks with technology and action. I had been trained to believe that I "delivered" a baby, even though healthy women push out their babies. Before that day it never occurred to me that a healthy woman having a normal labor wouldn't need my services, that there could be nothing to do—except give her room and stand by. But on that day my medical approach was superfluous. This event helped me understand that there needed to be a better balance of medicine and nature.

There is a biological as well as a psychological explanation for what I had just witnessed. The birthing woman's amazing transformation—her clarity of purpose and strength—was the result of the release of endorphins (naturally occurring hormones in the body that relieve pain and enhance the sense of overall well-being), basically acting like an internal dose of morphine without any of the risks or side effects. Athletes call the painkilling and euphoric effects of endorphins the "second wind" or "runner's high." It was the powerful sensations of childbirth itself that triggered her rush of endorphins. Her pride of achievement was also based in knowing that she was a capable woman. She had risen to the occasion, handled the physical challenges, and brought forth a new life.

Your project in reading this book is to create a flexible birth plan. My motivation in writing this book is to give you reliable facts about birth—based on the most up-to-date scientific evidence—that will enable you to design an experience that strikes a good balance between nature and human intervention. What practices are the safest? What practices are unnecessary? What practices are downright harmful? You deserve to have clear and objective answers. Only you can decide the right balance for you.

Childbirth hasn't changed since the beginning of history; only our attitudes and our methods ever change. Well-designed research studies reveal the truth behind attitudes and practices. With solid, reliable information in your hands, you have a better yardstick with which to evaluate everything related to your baby's impending birth: caregivers, institutions, practices, policies, and on-the-spot recommendations.

The Principles of Woman-Centered Childbirth

When it comes to childbirth, it is hard to improve upon the wisdom of nature. Science has shown in study upon study that the safest way for a healthy woman to give birth is naturally, with as few interventions as possible, because routine interventions can actually impede the body's natural birth processes. Technology, medications, and surgery are useful, even lifesaving, when certain types of serious complications arise; however, during normal labor a woman benefits more from the continuous presence of a skilled caregiver or companion who can help her navigate the difficult passages of labor. Watch and wait. These two actions are the key to safe and empowering maternity care. When nature is allowed to take its course, there is usually no reason to step in. Being patient and keeping a discerning eye open for signs of distress and for poor or good progress enables a pregnant woman's caregivers to give her the right kind and right amount of support.

Today, a woman can choose from among many different kinds of professional childbirth caregivers. (We'll talk about doctors, midwives, nurses, and doulas in this book.) A woman can choose from a variety of childbirth settings. (We'll talk about hospitals, out-of-hospital birth centers, and planned home births in this book.) The safest caregivers and the safest settings adopt an approach that lets the woman and her body—nature—determine the flow of labor support. An exception is a surgical birth.

Juliana Fehr, Ph.D., a midwife and coordinator of the nurse-midwifery program at Shenandoah University in Virginia, describes the interaction between a woman and her caregivers in an entirely woman-centered labor setting, "Birth is a dance and we're following the woman in labor. We dance around her. She's the most powerful person in the room because she's giving life. We stay back until we get the signs—the smell of amniotic fluid and other changes—and then the energy goes up in the room. She calls out to us." Fehr continues, "The mother has to feel safe in a trusting environment. She has to know she can scream or cry or do whatever she wants and it will be OK, she'll be loved. She's got to create the situation in which she will be nourished. She has to own the accomplishment of birth."

Heidi Rinehart, M.D., an obstetrician, gave birth under the care of a midwife. She agrees that birth must be woman centered. "Childbirth and welcoming a new baby into the world is a pivotal event in the life of a woman and a family. When a mom gives birth under her own power with the loving support of her family and the gentle guidance of a caregiver, it can be one of the most powerful, intimate, meaningful events in her life."

In 1996, the Coalition for Improving Maternity Services (CIMS) defined five philosophical keys that lead to the safest birth experiences:[1]

- Treating birth as a normal, natural process (not a disease)

- Exercising restraint and weighing scientific evidence before using drugs and other interventions (aka "First, do no harm")

- Empowerment of mothers and families

- Recognition of the autonomy of women

- Everyone—care providers, administrators, and pregnant women alike—assumes responsibility for their role in the birth process

Signs that you are receiving mother-friendly care include the following (these points are discussed in greater detail throughout the remainder of the book):[2]

- You should have unrestricted access to birth companions of your choice, including your spouse or partner, children, family members, and friends.

- You should have unrestricted access to *continuous* emotional and physical support from a woman skilled in childbirth, such as a doula or labor-support professional.

• You should have access to professional midwifery care if you want it.

• You should be provided accurate descriptive and statistical information about practices and procedures for birth care, including how often different interventions have been used in other births and their outcomes.

• Your care should be culturally competent—that is, sensitive and responsive to your specific ethnic and religious beliefs, values, and customs.

• You should have the freedom to walk, move about, and assume the positions of your choice during labor and birth (unless a restriction is specifically required to correct a complication), and you should never be placed lying flat on your back with your legs elevated (aka the lithotomy position).

• It should be clear to you what procedures your caregiver will use to collaborate and consult with other maternity services before the birth and if transfer from one birth site to another is necessary during labor, including how communication will be handled between your original caregiver and a second caregiver.

• A hospital, birth center, or caregiver should not *routinely* employ practices and procedures that are unsupported by scientific evidence, including but not limited to shaving, enemas, intravenous drips (IVs), withholding food and beverages, early rupture of membranes (aka the "bag of waters" or amniotic sac), and electronic fetal monitoring (EFM).

• A hospital or birth center should limit other interventions, including induction (artificially starting labor), episiotomy (surgical cutting to widen the vaginal opening for birth), and cesarean section.

• You should be provided with information about nondrug methods of pain relief.

- You should not feel that analgesic or anesthetic drugs are being promoted to you that are not specifically required to correct a complication.

- You should be permitted, even if you have a sick or premature newborn or an infant with congenital problems, to touch, hold, breastfeed, and care for your baby to the extent that's compatible with your condition.

- You should be provided with breastfeeding support and linked with appropriate community resources for postnatal support.

While the key element in a planned home birth is that you are in charge of the childbirth process and everything that happens to you, in a hospital you won't ever be in complete control. Having a choice about certain maternity care procedures is not the same as having autonomy, as doctors, nurse-midwives, and administrators in hospitals always retain the power to decide whether or not they will acquiesce to your choices. A doctor or hospital conceivably might try to pressure you to have a procedure you do not want. You are entitled to deny specific services. Similarly doctors are not required to do what you want if doing it goes against their professional judgment or preferences.

Worst-case scenario: If you disagree with hospital staff and fail in your attempts to negotiate your care to your satisfaction, your first option (other then complying) is to sign yourself out *against medical advice.* Of course, signing out of a hospital is not a tempting prospect in the midst of labor, but it is your legal right. Your second, and best, option is to navigate the legally mandated complaints procedures in the hospital to secure your wishes. (See chapter 13 for a detailed explanation of your legal rights.)

Best-case scenario: You have chosen a hospital or birth center that is overtly committed to woman-centered care. You are therefore receiving care from maternity-care providers and institutions where birth plans are welcomed and honored.

Planning as a Discovery Process

It is no secret that my goal in *Creating Your Birth Plan* is to support you in designing a safe and empowering birth that satisfies and delights you and your family. The best way I know to do that is to inform you about some of the issues you might wish to consider, point you toward good additional resources, teach you appropriate questions to ask, give you guidelines to measure the responses you get, and describe how to communicate your wishes to everyone involved in ways that medical professionals, personal advocates, institutions, and midwives alike will respect.

As I mentioned earlier in the introduction, I am suggesting that you plan for an event that is actually out of anyone's control. That sounds crazy. But, in fact, planning for birth can influence how well it goes. I am suggesting that you plan the process of birth, not a specific outcome. The vast majority of births do go more or less as planned. It is a good idea to build a degree of flexibility into your plan. I'll show you how later on.

I highly recommend keeping an informal journal as you read this book, and throughout your pregnancy, and use it to record your thoughts, feelings, and impressions about the different subjects you'll be introduced to as well as your direct experience of your condition and care. These thoughts will become the foundation of your written birth plan. At the end of the book, you'll learn how to draft the formal written plan that may be shared with your professional caregivers, if you so choose, but for the time being, any insights you have are for your own benefit. Use them to begin dialogues with your significant others and caregivers—to get feedback and elicit information.

Now, I must inform you that there are some people—including women's advocates—who believe that birth plans are adversarial documents and may "trigger" a doctor, midwife, or hospital staff to treat birthing women poorly. Hopefully not! But forewarned is forearmed. Evidence shows that planning produces safer outcomes.

To involve a reluctant male partner with you in planning, especially if he wants you just to do what a caregiver tells you without analysis, share the following metaphor with him. It should appeal to the masculine mind-set (it does to me). Think of all the care you would put into the process of buying a new car. You would look at the car's features, compare it to other vehicles, ask a lot of questions, and study the answers before settling on the vehicle that was right for you. Your baby's birth deserves even more attention.

Your birth plan is a tool for self-discovery. It can help steer your education about birth-related matters and foster communication with those who will support your labor. There is no single "correct" way to write a birth plan, just as there is no most appropriate way to effectively express yourself to doctors, midwives, nurses, hospitals, and birth centers. That being said, it's generally better when communication is an ongoing dynamic in a relationship rather than a frantic event that happens at the last possible moment.

Opportunities for Education and Open Communication

Interventions may become necessary at some point. Even in a natural birth, it is not always appropriate to avoid them completely. But if you are planning to give birth in a hospital, what can you do to guarantee that you won't be prey to the interventions of an overzealous obstetrician during your labor? Question your doctor every step of the way. A wonderful piece of research showed that when women simply asked, "Is that really necessary?" whenever an intervention was proposed during labor, the rate of unnecessary interventions that were being used dropped significantly.[3] "Are there any alternatives?" is another powerful question. Being well informed only increases your security.

Once you incorporate your research in a birth plan, discuss this plan with your birth attendants—obstetricians, nurses, midwives, and doulas, everyone—during your pregnancy. For instance, if you decide that you do not want an episiotomy, make it clear that this is your decision.

(Information on episiotomies is offered in chapter 8.) Since saying it once is sometimes not enough, you'd be smart to have it put in writing in your prenatal chart, and also for you to put it in your own handwriting, as an addition, when you sign the consent form that will be presented to you upon entering the hospital. This strategy is effective because it gives the message to your doctor and the hospital that you are really serious about your wishes, and it also reminds the hospital staff that they're vulnerable to litigation if your wishes as expressed are not followed. You can pick up the consent form from a hospital or birth center ahead of time, and then read and consider what it says at your leisure. Make any modifications, sign it, and bring it back to the hospital or birth center with you upon your admittance.

Here are a few suggestions of where and when you might discuss your birth plan with your caregivers.

- *Prenatal checkups.* Bring up the topics you want your birth plan to cover with your doctor or midwife—and any advocates like doulas— during your prenatal visits and explore them conversationally. What types of childbirth practices disturb or alarm you? Which aspects of care do you feel neutral about? Which aspects do you feel enthusiastic about?

    If you need more information about a technology, drug, or procedure, prenatal visits are great opportunities to ask. And if you want to more thoroughly understand your birth attendant's point of view about a technology, drug, and procedure, as well as its relevance to your situation, these are a good time for those discussions, too. As you casually dialogue, your wishes and opinions will be revealed to the caregiver.

- *A preliminary hospital visit.* When you're having a hospital birth, nurses are the key players in having a birth plan followed, as they will be looking in on you the most frequently. It's therefore a good idea to meet with the nursing staff ahead of time and get them on board with your birth plan. (Call ahead to choose a time to meet them when they expect the facility to be quieter.) If at all possible, there should be at least verbal agreement from the staff that the plan has been read and understood. Ideally the hospital's acknowledgment of your plan should come both from your doctor and from a nursing supervisor or a labor-and-delivery nurse, not just the admitting nurse. But because the doctor is responsible for supervising the efforts of the hospital's labor team, if you are a private patient, it is best if explicit acknowledgment comes from the doctor that he or she has read the plan and agrees to follow it and will ensure that any deviations from the plan are discussed with you before such actions are taken.

Find out what are the usual routines where you plan to give birth, and then, if you want to do it differently, decide if you really want to be a source of possible friction by doing it your way. If that item in your birth plan is truly important to you, such as "no routine electronic fetal monitoring," then you may want to change birth locations. When you're on-site, take a look around and determine if there's anything else that belongs in your plan or which you might need to bring in for your labor.

• *Adding the plan to your hospital/birth center files and chart prior to admission.* You are responsible for ensuring that your medical records are transported from your doctor's or midwife's office to the hospital or birth center prior to your arrival on the day (or night) of labor. Even if you're planning a home birth, it's an excellent practice to visit the hospital ahead of time just in case you end up one of the roughly 10 percent needing to be transferred to that hospital to give birth to your baby there. As I already said, stopping by gives you a chance to meet the labor-and-delivery nurses, head nurses, and administrators and share your birth plan with them.

• *On arrival at the hospital or birth center.* Make sure, again, that you have signed your birth plan and it has been attached to your chart. It needs to have been delivered with your medical records ahead of time. Bring along extra copies of the birth plan and hand them to every caregiver on staff who comes to work with you while you're in labor.

Your birth plan is a tool you can use to foster good communication and build understanding between you, your spouse or partner, and your caregivers. In the next chapter, we'll explore the stages of healthy childbirth, so you can begin planning for the birth of your child by imagining the best-case scenario.

Two

Best-Case Scenario

The Stages of Healthy Childbirth

"I was hoping for a natural birth," says Naomi. "My main preparation was reading about the stages of the delivery, so that I understood what would happen during the process. I wanted to know how to create positions that would make childbirth easier for me."

Most women's pregnancies and childbirths are normal and healthy. Mothers and babies come through them unharmed and go on to thrive. Family connections are strengthened. As long as we human beings have been around, so has natural—nontechnological and unmedicated—vaginal birth. Except for rare instances, the least amount of interference in the process of labor and birth is the best course of action that caregivers can suggest. A relaxed, well-informed woman who has taken good care of herself during pregnancy (getting adequate nutrition, rest, exercise, and making visits to a midwife or doctor), who then receives support throughout labor, and is given the privacy she requires to feel secure is most likely to have a safe and satisfying childbirth. With respectful support, she is able to navigate the stages and challenges of laboring and giving birth.

No doubt, the primary concern of everyone involved in childbirth is the ultimate health of a mother and her baby. But we've forgotten in our culture to let nature be our guide. The truth is that having babies is something that women *do,* and are biologically suited to do, rather than something that's being done *to* them. Above all else, during healthy labor pregnant women benefit from continuous one-on-one attendance of a midwife, a labor-and-delivery nurse, or a doctor. A doula, a family member, or a friend can provide emotional support and advocacy. When a woman feels in charge of her labor and understands that caring practitioners are there to support her needs, it enables her to relax and surrender to the process in which her body is engaged. Childbirth is a function of the female autonomic nervous system—like digestion or orgasm—so fear and stress impede its progress. Conversely, a sense of comfort and security eases the process.

Woman-centered childbirth, which can be defined as childbirth that puts all of the mother's needs above everyone else's, is shorter and less painful, and it produces fewer complications for mother and baby. All desired outcomes.

Your baby's birth should be an amazing and inspiring experience. Although the actual childbirth lasts only a short time, from a few hours to a couple of days, the birth doesn't stop when your baby emerges. Birth is not purely physiological, despite involving a significant physical event. Perhaps you dreamed about motherhood since you were a little girl or planned for years beforehand to get pregnant. Then, during nine months of gestation, you are contemplating the meaning of the event. Who will the baby be? Who will you, the mother, become? How will your life and relationships change? Once you're pregnant, already you've changed on a basic, primal level. You feel curious sensations in your abdomen, your sense of smell is heightened, and so forth. Afterward, you will probably look back on the birth experience and reflect on it. For better or for worse, it may color your view of the world and your personal capabilities. Thus, the influence of a child's birth has the potential to carry on for as long as you're alive and can remember.

In future chapters, we'll explore different factors that can contribute to the course and outcome of labor, along with various types of birth scenarios. But before we do, it is important for you to have a clear understanding of the stages of healthy labor—the kind that occurs without complications and is allowed to follow its natural progression. In other words, it doesn't involve drugs (which doctors use), medicinal herbs (which some midwives use), or instrumental and surgical interventions. Topics covered in this chapter will include helpful laboring positions, nourishment, and hydration.

Your Prenatal Care

We've chosen to limit this book to the actual process of labor and birth, although this book will be useful early on in your pregnancy or even before you're pregnant, at a time when you can make an informed plan. Everything you do during pregnancy leads up to the moment of birth. It is the culmination. Uneventful birth is an outcome of a healthy pregnancy.

During pregnancy your primary birth attendant (a doctor or midwife) will meet with you periodically to assess your health and the baby's health. Prenatal visits take place once a month from the second month of pregnancy on. In the first visit, the diagnosis of pregnancy is confirmed with a simple blood test. After the eighth month of pregnancy, the frequency of your visits increases to once a week. You are also given instructions to phone the doctor or midwife whenever you're worried about something. You don't have to wait for a prenatal visit to ask a question.

These prenatal visits are aimed at teaching you optimal health practices (such as nutrition, exercise, lifestyle, sexual behavior, limiting exposure to toxins), preventing complications, and the early detection of any deviations from normal. In a healthy pregnancy, you're not going to find deviations and there won't be complications. Your birth attendant will ask how you're doing, take your blood pressure, test your urine for protein, palpate your abdomen to measure the progress in the growth of your uterus and recommend vitamins, talk about nutrition and exercise, and basically send you home.

An important job of the caregiver is to offer you reassurance that you're OK. There is a powerful connection between the brain and uterus during pregnancy and childbirth. Stress and worry can be detrimental to the progress of your pregnancy. Hormones and brain chemicals influence pregnancy. You need to feel as relaxed and confident as possible. But this is not just a psychological issue. There is a biological element to the reassurance. It is indeed important to have your blood pressure taken to determine if it's high and your urine checked for protein, as these are signs of preeclampsia. It's important that your belly is palpated to be sure the uterus is growing at an appropriate rate and to confirm that you're not having twins instead of a singleton baby. Late in pregnancy, you want to be sure the baby is not in a breech, or feetfirst, position, and so forth. There are numerous valid reasons for regular biological checking.

Another major purpose of prenatal care is education about what to expect and watch out for both during the pregnancy and the birth. For women between the ages of fifteen and forty-five, in 75 or 80 percent of cases you can certainly expect there to be no problems. Your prenatal meetings with your birth attendant are your opportunity to create a birth plan, ask the type of questions that occur throughout this book, and find out as much as you can about yourself, your birth attendant, and the care facility.

Prenatal visits also allow you to get to know and develop trust in your primary healthcare provider. That way, when this individual comes into your room during labor, your nervous system immediately recognizes the birth attendant as a "friend" and "ally." In the current hospital maternity-care system, everyone else who is present during your birth most likely will be a stranger. When you see the familiar caregiver, you'll feel reassured because someone knows you and your body, your needs, and your wishes.

So, let's say you have sailed through all that. Now labor is imminent.

What Is Labor?

The uterus is a large, circular muscle lying in a woman's lower abdominal cavity next to her intestines. Inside the uterus is a lined cavity that during pregnancy holds a fetus (the baby inside the womb). The fetus floats in a sack of clear liquid called amniotic fluid. It is attached by a cord (the umbilical cord) to the placenta, which is attached to the lining of the uterus. Blood vessels inside the cord carry oxygen and nutrients from the mother's placenta to the fetus, and carry waste from the fetus back through the placenta to the mother's body. On the lower end of the uterus, there is an opening (the cervix) that has a strong sphincter muscle around it to hold it closed so that the fetus won't fall out before it is ready to be born.

In order for a baby to be born, the uterus contracts over and over again, and pushes the fetus against the cervix, which then gradually opens wide to a diameter of ten centimeters, or about four inches. Then the uterine muscle must continue to contract in order to squeeze the baby through the cervix, down the vagina—which is able to stretch wide enough to accommodate the fetus—and out into the world. That's labor.

By definition, labor is the intermittent contracting of the uterus to push the fetus out of a woman's body. Active labor can take from an hour to a couple of days. It has three stages. Sometimes it is gentle, and other times it is intense. Your caregivers don't have to watch the clock and worry about the duration of each stage as long as every sign indicates that you and your baby are OK. This is a theme we're going to repeat throughout the book.

The Natural Progression of Labor

When does labor normally start? A pregnant woman's "due date" is calculated at forty weeks past conception as determined by using ultrasound readings of her uterus and/or the date of her last menstrual period. Forty weeks is an average length based on the range of possible lengths of gestation, meaning that any time two weeks before or two weeks after that due date would also be perfectly normal.

Near the end of pregnancy, the uterus, which is now stretched quite large, will from time to time have prelabor contractions called Braxton Hicks contractions. These contractions are intermittent and perfectly normal, yet they are not true labor. With true labor, contractions are no longer intermittent, but become regular every few minutes.

As to what starts labor, you may be surprised to learn that no one knows the scientific reason. We know something about the mechanism of labor once it starts, but not what triggers it in the first place. Once labor starts up, the brain sends hormones to the uterus that control the ongoing contractions. As I mentioned, labor is a function of the autonomic nervous system. Like breathing and digestion, a woman has no conscious control over it. Truly, she can only create an environment that supports it, and then go along for the "ride" and respond as flexibly as she can to unfolding developments.

Whenever you believe labor has started, you should pick up the telephone and have a conversation about what you are experiencing with your obstetrician, midwife, or the office nurse or hospital staff, and find out whether or not they think it's OK or concerning. You are doing your healthcare provider a favor by opening a line of communication, alerting him or her to your situation, and getting any advice you need. Often the care provider says, "It sounds good; if all continues to go well, come in when you are having contractions every five minutes." He or she might mention specific signs to watch out for. So, an initial plan is created.

For the early hours of labor it is OK for you to be alone—alone, but not out of touch. It would be helpful to have a partner, neighbor, relative, or some human being in the house with you at this point to assist you in case something suddenly goes wrong. During early labor you can rest quietly at home before you go to the hospital for care or before you have a midwife arrive on your doorstep. Many care providers recommend that you drink a glass of wine, eat a small meal, and lie down. You're going to need all your strength later on, so it's a good idea to conserve it.

The First Stage of Labor

Stage one of labor is the period of time during which the uterus contracts and pushes the fetus against the cervix, gradually opening it up. The cervix is, by necessity, a very strong muscle, and it takes a lot of pushing to open it up—more so if it is the first birth. This stage is a slow process, taking many hours, and it is important that it go fairly slowly, as the mother's body must be given a chance to soften and stretch wide open so she won't be harmed. The process is also slow because the baby is moving down the "birth canal" through a large hole, or opening, formed by the mother's pelvic bone. The pelvic bone is shaped like a bowl with a circular opening in the bottom. Pushing the baby through this hole is important because it squeezes amniotic fluid—the "water"—out of the baby's lungs so that the lungs are empty and ready to be filled up with air when the baby has been born and takes its first breath. If this rhythmic squeezing of the lungs does not occur, such as when a cesarean section is done, the baby has a much harder time getting its respiration going after birth, and there is an increased risk of a serious condition known as respiratory distress syndrome (see page 140).

Sometimes the baby's head is slightly larger than the hole in the mother's pelvic bone. During stage one of labor, the baby's head is gradually "molded" by contractions so it can fit through. A baby's skull is not a single bone but a bunch of bones fitted together like a jigsaw puzzle. They are softer than adult bones, as they're not yet calcified. If the baby's head were round, the circumference would be too large for the hole in the mother's pelvic bone. But the skull can be molded. When slowly pushed over a period of hours, the shape of the skull will change without damaging the brain. Part of what the contractions do is move the baby's head into the pelvis and alter its shape.

It is important that the molding of the head take place gradually so as not to put undue pressure on the baby's brain and possibly cause brain damage. The baby's head quickly returns to a normal shape after birth and, if the labor has not been rushed, no damage will have been done.

When should you go to the hospital? It depends on several factors, including how long it will take you to get to the hospital, whether or not this is your first baby (in which case your labor usually will take considerably longer), how comfortable you are staying at home and waiting for a little while without panicking, and if there's someone else around. If you rush to the hospital at the first sign of a contraction, it is likely you will be sent home—a frustrating and anticlimactic occurrence. Time your contractions for a while. If they are regular, and you have two or more in a ten-minute period, then it is probably time to go in. Call the hospital first and check with the admitting nurse or midwife. Ask his or her advice. Staying home during the early hours of labor has the advantage of resulting in fewer unnecessary interventions.[1] It has the disadvantage, if you are nervous, of potentially triggering you to feel anxiety.

It is crucial that the contractions of the uterus are intermittent with a break in between. This is because the baby gets its oxygen and other important nutrients from the mother through the umbilical cord. In order for oxygen and nutrients to get to the cord, they must first pass through the wall of the uterus and into the placenta. But when the uterus is contracting, it squeezes so hard that it is impossible for anything to get through the uterine wall, and so the supply of oxygen is temporarily cut off from the baby. Only during the breaks between contractions can oxygen and other vital nutrients pass through the uterine wall to the placenta and then through the cord to the baby.

A doctor or midwife can determine your baby's status and level of distress by listening to your baby's heartbeat with a fetal stethoscope (fetoscope) between your contractions. People debate how frequently to listen, but everyone agrees that it should be monitored from time to time. Even the American College of Obstetricians and Gynecologists (ACOG) concurs that a fetoscope is as effective as an electronic fetal monitor.[2] The purpose is to ensure that the baby's heart rate is neither too high nor too low, to make sure the baby is tolerating everything well. Your caregiver can monitor your status and level of distress by checking your blood pressure, pulse, color, respiration, and alertness.

Uterine contractions vary in intensity and they can be painful. This phenomenon, which is commonly referred to as labor pain, is an essential component of childbirth, as it creates a feedback mechanism that stimulates the brain to send hormones to the uterus that move labor and birth along. When there are no sensations like these, as happens when women are given nerve-blocking medications like epidurals, the process of labor can slow down and even stop. For this reason, many caregivers prefer to adopt measures that help women handle the intensity of the experience without stopping it.

Every intervention has the potential to initiate a cascade of consequences, and therefore the merits of each must be considered carefully before it is done.

The Second Stage of Labor

A transition occurs as the laboring woman shifts from stage one to stage two of labor. When her uterine contractions have pushed a woman's softened cervix completely open to a diameter of ten centimeters (about four inches), the baby is now ready to move the rest of the way down through the vagina and opening of the pelvic bone and come out through the vaginal opening into the world. This passage is the second stage of labor.

From the point of view of someone standing in the delivery room, the most dramatic thing that announces stage two is the sudden need of the birthing woman to "push" the baby out of her body by bearing down hard. Again, this is a reflexive action of the nervous system over which she has no control. Her body does this of its own accord when the time is right.

In days gone by, it was formerly believed that it was sometimes a good thing to tell the woman *not* to push—for instance, if the doctor hadn't arrived yet—but we now know that the woman must be allowed to push when her body tells her to. If you were nauseated and about to vomit, there would be nothing in the world that could stop you from heaving. The impulse to push is just as powerful. Trying to slow down labor at this stage in the progression, perhaps so the doctor has time to rush over, is a real mistake, as a complicated set of responses are taking place in the woman's body at this point in time, and these responses are finely tuned to bring the baby safely out of her body.

Birth attendants should be giving you encouragement during stage two. Your midwife, partner, or doctor does best when making supportive statements, such as, "You're doing well," "That's good," and, "Go for it!" No one should ever push down on the abdomen in an attempt to forcibly move the baby along. Someone may also take a mirror and hold it between your legs so you can see the baby's head or hair. In this stage, when the baby's head is crowning, and it's pushing out through your perineum, the head is visible to everyone who is there. It is a truly miraculous and awesome sight.

There is also an important reason not to rush labor during the second stage. The opening of the vagina must stretch big enough to let the baby's head pass through and on out. The baby's head is the largest part of the baby, so when the opening has stretched wide enough to let the head pass through, the rest of the baby follows easily and quickly. This stretching of the vagina must take place slowly so as to significantly decrease the chance that the vagina will tear during the process of stretching. If the baby's head is allowed to slowly pass on out, there will, in fact, be little or no tearing. If the second stage is hurried, however, there is more likely to be tearing. This is why, until recently, many doctors would cut the vagina open wider. Now we know this is not necessary.

When a laboring woman pushes, her baby's head bulges out, and when the contraction is over, the head retracts a little bit. With every push and bulge, the perineum is stretched until it finally opens. A woman's bones and tissues are built in order to let babies out, as long as enough time is allowed for opening. Normally, the structure of the bones is not an issue as long as a woman has received decent nutrition in her lifetime.

Previously, many doctors and hospitals thought that the second stage of labor should not last longer than two hours. They were fearful that the baby might not get enough air, so when the allotted two hours was up they would jump in and try to pull the baby out. We now know the time limit on the second stage of labor was a mistake and that, as long as the mother and baby are doing OK, there should never be a time limit put on the second stage of labor. Particularly with a first baby, the second stage can normally last many hours without difficulty.

Many of the most extreme interventions in contemporary labor are ultimately used as a result of doctors' impatience with the progression of birth. It is common for hospitals to establish rules about how long the second stage may last before a doctor is required to take an action. Be mindful that these rules often extend to birth centers located within the confines of a hospital, too, even though a nurse-midwife is attending the labor. Excellent scientific research, however, shows that watching the clock is a big mistake. So long as a woman and her baby are in good condition and there are signs of progress, elapsed time is an arbitrary reason to hurry.[3]

At some point during the last several weeks of gestation, the baby settles into the pelvis, hopefully in a head-down position. If it does not, an attempt may be made by caregivers to turn the baby. The baby's head is also rotating in stage two. As the baby comes down the birth canal, the baby's face turns and lines up with the pelvis. There are differences in the diameter of certain features on the head, and as the head turns, the baby gradually finds the path of least resistance. In general, the baby's head is positioned facing either toward the spine or the front.

By the time the baby is ready to pop out, it is in a different position than it was in the first stage. There has been a change in the shape of the baby's head, a change in the position of the baby's head, its lungs have been wrung out, and the mother's cervix, vagina, and perineum have stretched. All of these changes take time.

The Third Stage of Labor

When the baby has been born—that is, fully out of the vagina—the baby is still attached to the umbilical cord, which, as you already know, runs up the vagina into the uterus where it is attached to the placenta. Some people used to think it important to quickly cut this cord, but science has shown that the opposite is true. The umbilical cord pulsates and pumps blood into the baby, and this is important blood, sort of like a final transfusion. So it is best to wait until the cord stops pulsating, which usually takes a few minutes, and then to cut the cord.

At the moment of birth, the baby takes a breath and the lungs expand, so, from then, the baby can breathe on its own. Since the baby has never tried to breathe through its nose and mouth before, however, sometimes there may be secretions in the nose and mouth interfering. These can be easily removed.

When the baby is out and the cord is still attached, if the doctor or midwife believes the baby may have lacked sufficient oxygen during birth, blood can be withdrawn from the umbilicus and sent to a lab to test it for chemical changes and oxygenation.

Good scientific research has shown that a baby should be immediately handed to the mother and never be taken from her from birth onward.[4] Many essential processes, both in the baby and mother, take place in the first few minutes after birth. Having the mother hold the baby during this time greatly facilitates these processes. The baby needs to be checked out briefly. Placing the baby on the mother's abdomen and chest keeps it warm during the exam. Not only does this allow the mother to watch and learn, it also helps her more quickly bond with her new baby.

All babies are given a score (an Apgar) based on breathing, heart rate, muscle tone, reflex irritability, and skin color. Each measure is assigned different points. A perfect score is ten points. The Apgar is taken at one minute, five minutes, and ten minutes after birth. If the skin is tinted blue at birth, indicating oxygen deprivation, the infant might get a seven- or eight-point rating. But if the skin pinks up by minute five or minute ten, and its rating goes up to ten, the infant is considered perfectly healthy.

The mother also needs to put the baby to her breast at this time, as her breasts are full of special fluid called colostrum, which contains large amounts of important nutrients designed by nature for the newborn. These nutrients include vital antibodies that give the baby immunity to many dangerous germs. It is also important to remember that the breast only makes milk if the milk is taken from it; so putting the baby on the breast first thing helps to get milk production going. A few minutes after the baby's birth, the placenta detaches itself from the woman's uterus and comes out through her vagina, usually along with a small amount of blood. With this, stage three ends, and the birth is complete.

There is a small but real risk of hemorrhage in stage three. As the placenta detaches from the uterine lining, it leaves behind a raw area where its blood vessels used to connect. The only reason why a woman normally doesn't hemorrhage is that the uterus immediately clamps down once the baby is out. This stops the exposed vessels from bleeding. Breastfeeding stimulates this response. It is common practice to give the woman an injection to facilitate this clamping-down process. Both midwives and doctors may give injections of a drug called oxytocin, which is sometimes used for labor inducement (see chapter 6 for more details). The hemorrhage that results from the failure of the uterus to clamp down may be the result of uterine exhaustion or overstimulation of the uterus with inducing or augmenting drugs.

The action of the uterus also pushes the placenta out. The passage of the placenta, or afterbirth, out of the vagina is spontaneous and usually takes place within about fifteen minutes.

A woman who just gave birth needs someone with her during this last piece of childbirth. Good birth attendants stand and watch. Once stage three is complete, it's better if a woman who has had a home birth is not alone, as she might need someone to make a phone call for her. But she no longer needs professional assistance.

You can read more about your baby's initial evaluation and treatment in chapter 11, "Welcome to the World! Baby-Friendly Hospital Care."

Helpful Laboring Positions

Women's bodies are best positioned for giving birth when they are standing, sitting, or squatting—in other words, *vertical* laboring positions. Horizontal laboring positions, and specifically lying flat on the back, are the worst possible positions in which to give birth. Horizontal positions, including a semi-reclining position, put tremendous weight on the tailbone, press the baby's head against the mother's aorta (the big artery that supplies blood to the placenta), thus decreasing the blood supply to nourish the baby, force the mother to give birth "uphill"

against gravity, and decrease the size of the pelvic outlet, making it harder for a woman to push out the baby.

When enough obstetricians finally acknowledged that a horizontal position was detrimental, they set about designing a variety of adjustable beds and chairs. All such devices are mechanical, made of metal, quite complex—allowing for a number of positions. You can use them to elevate your feet or your head, lie on your side with one leg elevated, and more. Or you may opt for a simpler contraption, such as a beanbag chair, a special wooden birthing stool, or a chair that has curved seats, rounded edges, and built-in handholds to help you apply leverage without falling off.

While a vertical position is the key to an easier and safer labor, mobility is the key to a comfortable one. You have an innate sense of what's happening inside your body. As your baby moves around during labor and as you move to accommodate the changes in pressure and sensation, you will actually be facilitating your labor.

Every baby and mother fit together in a unique physiological way. While the stages of labor are experienced in common, you may prefer one position over another. Some mothers prefer to be on their hands and knees, others to stand upright with a partner, doula, or whomever standing supporting you from behind. Or a laboring woman might choose to bend forward over a birth ball, squat and lean forward, or lie on her side. There are advantages to each position:

Squatting: Opens the pelvic outlet and takes advantage of gravity. May require less bearing down, and may enhance the baby's rotation and descent.

Semi-reclining: A good resting position that takes some advantage of gravity. It is more useful for vaginal exams and less useful for pushing.

Sitting upright: Another good resting position that takes some advantage of gravity. It is a useful position for getting a back rub. If you sit on a birthing stool, or on a toilet, instead of a springy birth ball, you'll have a firmer surface to push against.

Hands and knees: May help relieve backache by bringing the baby forward, but it is basically gravity neutral. It assists in the rotation of the baby from a posterior position.

Lying on your side: A good resting position, it may slow a very rapid labor, as it is gravity neutral, and therefore may be helpful in avoiding tearing.

Underwater birthing: Underwater birthing means the baby emerges from the mother while the mother is sitting in a large tub of warm water. It is designed to ease a baby's transition from the womb to the world. According to the scientific evidence, this kind of birth is a perfectly safe choice for those who wish to experience it with one proviso: There needs to be a trained birth attendant on hand.[5]

A few procedures can interfere with a woman's mobility during labor. Lines inserted in a vein for hydration and the electrodes connected with electronic fetal monitoring devices impede motion, and so do epidural catheters—not to mention the fact that epidurals temporarily paralyze the laboring woman from the waist down. In a natural-birth scenario, at home or in an out-of-hospital birth center, none of these procedures would be involved. But they are very common in hospital-birth scenarios.

Nourishment and Hydration

The scientific evidence shows that you need food and beverages during labor to keep your strength up and to energize you, and also to make you feel better.[6] Of course, you don't need to make yourself eat unless you feel hungry. But if you are hungry, you should eat! You might want to plan to have small snacks around to munch on intermittently. Think of yourself as an athlete who needs calories to succeed. You should drink whatever you enjoy drinking. You'll need to take in lots of liquids because you'll be perspiring like crazy for several hours.

Labor is comparable to running a marathon. It's called labor because you're working hard. It is quite normal for women to urinate frequently during labor. If you were to read the electronic fetal monitor strips in a hospital, you would find many gaps in them for this reason.

Some hospitals don't allow women in labor to eat and drink because all the women—not just the ones with complications—are being treated like surgical patients. In these cases, women in labor are usually given an IV for hydration. The idea behind withholding food and beverages is that you may vomit during surgery and aspirate the contents of your stomach into your lungs. Today we know that this is not a real risk during childbirth. Normal childbirth is *not* a surgical procedure. The only reason to have an IV is if you're throwing up and not tolerating fluids.

You may be offered ice chips. While this is a nice gesture, it is an inadequate source of hydration. You'll need more fluids and food than that to keep up your energy. You're going to be doing a whole lot of hard work when your baby is ready to emerge. Hopefully your hospital will allow you to eat and drink freely during your labor. If you're working with a midwife at home or in the hospital, this won't be an issue.

Good reasons to withhold food and drink:

• You are on your way to get a cesarean section.

• There are serious signs of fetal or maternal distress.

Adding Your Wishes to Your Birth Plan

Now that you're armed with knowledge of a normal, healthy birth, you'll be able to use the knowledge to begin evolving a personalized birth plan as you read through the remainder of the book. At the end of chapter 1, you were invited to begin a journal. I suggest you turn to your journal now and spend a few minutes jotting down some notes on your current impressions, thoughts, and feelings about the three stages of birth.

As you daydream, you may want to involve your partner or to get feedback from a close and trusted friend. Maybe you have questions to ask a care provider. Note them. It's nice to have a record of ideas and inspiration as a clear reminder of what you want to say.

In each stage of labor, different kinds of natural and high-tech coping strategies are available. You'll read about tools and techniques in later chapters. For now, what's your sense of your ideal birth if everything were to go perfectly? Normal birth is more statistically reasonable to anticipate than complicated birth, so it's good to plan for it.

One of the first things you'll begin to consider as you develop your birth plan is where to have your baby. This decision goes hand in hand with the selection of your primary maternity caregiver. In the next chapter, we'll explore different birth locations. Your wishes for how to handle the onset of labor and early labor, and then manage active labor and pushing out your baby are closely related to your decision of birth site.

Three

Selecting Your Birth Location

Do You Want to Have Your Baby in a Hospital,
an Out-of-Hospital Birth Center, or at Home?

"I wanted to have my baby in a hospital so I would feel free to scream and be loud; I didn't want to disturb the neighbors in my apartment building."

"The main reason I wanted a home birth is that I educated myself as much as possible on what would be a safe, gentle birth for the baby that also would give me the opportunity to labor in a relaxed atmosphere. That seemed the best way to have a great birth, for the baby to come easily, and for my husband and me to enjoy the process, rather than being afraid. I wanted it to be an amazing, life-transforming event."

"We visited several birth centers and fell in love with the atmosphere in the birth center where I ultimately had my baby. There was something wonderful about the way the team of midwives interacted with us and with each other that impressed us. It was also closer to the hospital than our house, and I felt reassured knowing that in case of trouble I wouldn't have to travel far."

"Frankly, I didn't give it much consideration. I gave birth in a hospital because it seemed the logical place to do that. Everyone I know went to the hospital. My doctor is excellent and the nurses there treated us as if we were their own family."

These are the voices of real women describing how they chose a birth location. In creating your birth plan, the most fundamental decision you will make is where to give birth. Why does it matter if you labor in a hospital, an out-of-hospital (freestanding) birth center, or at home? Birth location dictates the choice of your primary caregiver—either a midwife or an obstetrician—and the kind of assistance that this practitioner is able to provide to you.

Here, we'll explore the pros and cons of having a baby in a hospital, an out-of-hospital birthing center, or at home, as well as the caregiver and assistance options available in each. How can you determine whether or not these environments are mother friendly? The purpose of this chapter is to lay a foundation for your birth plan. As you read on and learn more information in later chapters about what typically happens in different types of care settings and under the supervision of different types of caregivers, you may wish to return to this chapter and reevaluate your initial decision.

Understanding Hospital Birth

More than 90 percent of planned births in America occur in hospitals.[1] Interestingly, in this setting women have the least autonomy of any possible environment during labor, while they often *feel* the greatest sense of security. (Whether or not they actually *are* safer is a different matter altogether, and something that you must purposefully assess on a case by case basis.) The biggest advantage of hospital birth is that if anything goes seriously wrong, a woman is already near a surgeon. Obstetricians are surgeons. If you have a truly high-risk medical condition, you'd be wise to have your baby in a hospital. At some hospitals you may choose to be attended either by a midwife or an obstetrician.

Another advantage to hospital birth is that it gives you access to technology and greater access to drugs. In many hospitals, drugs and various forms of technology are considered part of the routine. You may even feel pressured to use them. But you may also feel more emotionally secure. Last, in a hospital you can escape the routine duties of your home life—there are no dishes in the sink to wash, no children to tend, and so forth. When you're laboring or recuperating from labor, it's nice to take it easy.

What Happens When You Arrive at the Hospital?

During the planning phase of a healthy pregnancy, if you're like most women you'll arrange to visit the hospital. That way, on your due date you'll be at least semi-familiar with the facilities and admission procedures. You'll want to look at the labor rooms, surgical rooms, and waiting rooms for your family members. You may meet with one or more of the labor-and-delivery nurses. Often hospitals have special birthing rooms that include hot tubs, rocking chairs, and other extras. You might want to visit these. Maternity services are a top moneymaker for hospitals and doctors, and there is enormous competition. Most hospitals put together a comprehensive pitch, with lavish brochures and tours, to attract consumers. When you are selecting your birth location, you're in the driver's seat, except in remote communities where there is only one hospital.

Let's say you have chosen to go the hospital route. What happens once you're in labor? The first place you go is admissions to fill out forms and provide billing information. It is your responsibility to ensure that your prenatal records have been forwarded from your doctor's office to the hospital ahead of time, so they will be there when you arrive. The staff needs to know what went on during your pregnancy as this influences what is and isn't done during labor and birth. Your doctor won't be there when you arrive, and if you are working with an in-hospital midwife, she may or may not be there yet. The other people who took care of you outside the hospital, such as office nurses, don't work there. So if there are important things to know, like that you're allergic to penicillin—whatever it is—you've got to inform the hospital staff.

You must specifically request that your prenatal-care provider forward a copy of your birth plan to the hospital with your records, but bring extra copies along anyhow.

Basic information is requested even if your records are present. Admissions personnel ask questions from a checklist designed so hospital staff can determine your history at a glance. It's an attempt to overcome any communication gaps between your prenatal-care providers and your childbirth-care providers. You may be asked questions that weren't asked during pregnancy. For instance, in some hospitals nurses ask questions to get a handle on your tolerance for pain. This is important. If you give them a false impression, or you are misevaluated, you might not get the kind of help you need—you could get too much or too little. Another question you are likely to be asked is whether or not you plan to breastfeed.

The admitting nurse takes your history and does a physical assessment, including a vaginal exam. The point is to determine how well labor is progressing by inserting fingers inside your vagina and feeling how dilated your cervix is and how far the baby has descended. After doing this, the nurse might say you're not in labor and send you home. A lot of women get sent home. Or she may put you on an electronic fetal monitor for a few minutes to evaluate your contractions and make sure you really are in labor.

Then the nurse asks you to sign a release form. Part of her job is to elicit your fully informed consent. Consent forms have two purposes: to protect you and to protect the hospital. Your permission is needed for them to do things to you. You are saying it's OK and agreeing that you cannot sue them—although in reality signing such routine forms does not prevent you from any future actions. The hospital's motive is to avoid litigation. But you also need to be provided with information on the pros and cons of what will be done to you so that you can make an informed choice. You need to be fully informed about the possible benefits and risks of all planned interventions. Should the need for additional procedures arise you may be asked to sign other consent forms.

It is important for you to know that you are in control of this process. You don't have to sign anything until you are satisfied with the explanation you receive. A hospital cannot kick you out if you won't sign their release form. First of all, it would be bad public relations to refuse to admit a woman in active labor. Secondly, there is a federal law known as the Emergency Medical Treatment and Active Labor Act (EMTALA) that requires hospitals to admit women in active labor or be fined.[2] During the admissions process, having a written birth plan can be very important. Unless you specifically checked ahead of time that it was forwarded to the hospital with your prenatal records, your birth plan will only be attached to your hospital chart when you arrive. This greatly facilitates admissions, as the admitting nurse can read the birth plan and answer nine out of ten questions already.

By law, you are not required to sign the hospital's consent form. You can refuse to sign it. You also have the option of customizing the form by putting a line through any listed procedure and attaching a list of procedures that you specifically refuse. Sign the form and be sure to place your initials beside your changes. Documenting your refusal formally protects the hospital from potential litigation for *not* doing a procedure. For your convenience, pick up the form ahead of time. You may file it with the hospital up to thirty days early—but no more. For additional information about consent forms and different state regulations you may encounter, contact or visit the websites of maternal advocacy groups, such as Birth Policy and the International Cesarean Awareness Network (see Resources).

Upon admission in active labor, your street clothes are taken away and you are given a hospital gown. They put you in a wheelchair and wheel you to the maternity ward or your private room. You are essentially turned into a "patient." Of course, you can assert yourself and say, "I'm walking to my room," if you would prefer it.

Who can accompany you into labor and who can't? Hospital policies about companions during labor vary by institution. Fifty years ago, even fathers were asked to wait outside. Today, there is almost not a hospital left where you are forbidden to bring a spouse or partner, mother, or sister— at least one person close to you. So, you'll need to ask ahead of time about the elements of the birth experience that are important to you.

Valuable Questions for Hospitals

While most hospitals work to ensure a high standard of care, you may experience certain procedures in hospitals that run counter to scientific evidence and counter to the signs of mother-friendly care that we looked at in chapter 1 (see pages 11–13), such as limitations on visitors and visiting hours, routine intravenous fluids, routine withholding of food and drink, limitations on moving around freely and on laboring positions, routine electronic fetal monitoring for low-risk women, and not allowing your new baby to be with you at all times. We'll talk about each of these items in later chapters.

How can you find out if the institutional policies of a hospital conflict with your decisions about your care? Ask. Try the following questions:

- At what point do you recommend that I come to the hospital?

- How soon after I come to the hospital will my primary healthcare provider see me?

- How much time can I expect my primary healthcare provider to spend with me during labor?

- If I write a birth plan, will it be honored and will it go in my hospital chart?

- How often are vaginal exams performed during labor?

- Are showering and bathing allowed during labor for pain relief?

- Does this hospital allow underwater births? What facilities are available for underwater births?

- How many people are allowed to be with me during labor and childbirth?

- How many people are allowed to be with me if there is a need for cesarean section?

- What is the hospital's policy regarding children attending the birth?

• Are eating and drinking allowed during labor?

• What laboring positions are recommended and/or allowed?

• Is videotaping allowed?

• Can my partner cut the umbilical cord?

• Can my baby stay in the room with me?

• How long will I be able to stay in the hospital after my baby is born?

• Can I leave earlier if I want?

The answers to these questions will help you determine if a hospital birth is right for you and your baby.

Understanding Out-of-Hospital Birth Centers

Out-of-hospital birth centers are a place in the community where a low-risk woman can choose to go to give birth. They are not, in most cases, owned and operated by a hospital but rather by a group of midwives and/or an organization of women. In general, midwives manage births that take place in out-of-hospital birth centers, and women have greater freedom and birth options in birth centers than they do in hospitals. But are they as safe as hospitals? For low-risk pregnancies, the evidence says yes. In case of an emergency, a midwife at the birth center usually consults with a doctor by phone to decide whether or not to transport the woman to the hospital. Obstetricians are affiliated with an out-of-hospital birth center for exactly this reason—to be available for consultation when necessary—and some states legally require birth centers to have these affiliations. Birth centers are very safe because they are purposefully located close enough to hospitals to get there in less than half an hour. That's the average time it takes to prepare an operating room for a cesarean.

The biggest difference between a hospital and a birth center is in the woman-centered orientation. Women can have a birth managed according to their preferences. In a birth center, you are unlikely to have food or beverages withheld from you. You can have as many companions as you want, including children, extended family, and friends. In a birth center, attendants are trained to assist in many kinds of natural birth. Upon arrival in a birth center, you may be asked to sign a consent form, but it is unlikely to be as elaborate as in a hospital.

A birth center differs from a hospital in its routine laboring practices and use of interventions. In birth centers, your labor won't be induced with drugs, and although they have access to labor-augmenting drugs like Pitocin, such drugs are more conservatively used than in hospitals. IV fluids are available, as is electronic fetal monitoring; however, these are also rarely employed. At clear signs of fetal distress, you will be transferred to a hospital. Forceps and vacuum extractors are available, but rarely used.

As in a hospital, a birth-center birth liberates a woman from the demands of home, but the environment does not "medicalize" her condition. You'll have one-on-one continuous care not available in the hospital. Your unique cultural beliefs and needs will be honored. Emotionally, the surroundings are designed to be much less stressful and less startling to your sensibilities and provide more structure than you probably have at home.

Valuable Questions for Birth Centers

When you visit a birth center for evaluation, the questions are similar to those you'd ask on your tour of a hospital. Try these:

- At what point do you recommend that I come to the birth center?

- How soon after I come to the birth center will my primary health-care provider see me?

- How much time can I expect my healthcare provider to spend with me during labor?

- If I write a birth plan, will it be honored?

- How often are vaginal exams performed during labor?

- Are showering and bathing allowed during labor?

- Does this center allow underwater births? What facilities are available for underwater births?

- How many people are allowed to be with me during labor and delivery?

- What is the birth center's policy regarding children attending the birth?

- Are eating and drinking allowed during labor?

- What laboring positions are recommended and/or permitted?

- Is videotaping allowed?

- Can my partner cut the umbilical cord?

- Can my baby stay in the room with me?

- How long will I be able to stay in the birth center after my baby is born?

- Can I leave earlier if I want?

The answers to these questions will help you decide if a birth center is right for you and your baby.

Understanding Home Birth

Planned out-of-hospital births, under the care of trained midwives, have been proven to be as safe a birth option for a woman with a low-risk pregnancy as hospitals.[3] It is important to distinguish between planned and unplanned out-of-hospital birth locations.[4] When a baby arrives in a taxicab on the way to the hospital, it is an accidental, *unplanned* out-of-hospital birth. When a midwife catches a baby in a woman's bedroom, it is a *planned* out-of-hospital birth. The former is not as safe as the latter. In this section, we are discussing the latter, *planned* type of scenario.

With a home birth, a woman is in her own territory in familiar settings and is in control of who is there and what is done. Her family, including her children, can be with her. Low-risk childbirth doesn't require hospital paraphernalia, such as electronic fetal monitors, X-rays, gowns, masks, special beds for the women, and special tables for the baby. The vagina is not sterile and the baby is not sterile after coming through the vagina, so a sterile surgical field is not necessary for childbirth. The midwife can bring to the home everything that is necessary for low-risk, normal birth and for the management of most complications, including oxygen, sterile wipes, Pitocin, and a fetal stethoscope.

The notion that "nothing can be done in the home if trouble comes" is a myth. Home-birth midwives can successfully manage most complications and they know when it is necessary to transfer a woman to a hospital. Some complications, such as when a baby's head is born but the shoulders get stuck, require no special equipment whatsoever, only a skilled birth attendant's hands. These are just as well managed at home as in the hospital.

Home birth is the most private and woman-centered birth location available, and under the care of a trained midwife, planned home birth is actually safer than hospital birth, for a number of reasons. First, natural birth is safer than medical birth because women are more relaxed—their more tranquil state allows the release of a set of hormones that initiate and regulate normal, physiological labor and birth. These hormones are often in short supply in women giving birth in hospitals. In unfamiliar settings, women often experience anxiety and fear, which release a different set of hormones that interfere with normal labor. During home birth, as no time pressure is involved, women's bodies open gradually and have time to soften and stretch to make room for the baby to emerge relatively peacefully.

Second, women have already been exposed to the germs that inhabit their own home environments. They have antibodies against these germs and have already given their immunity to these germs to the babies inside their wombs. Having a home birth eliminates the risk of infection from exposure to unfamiliar bacteria or viruses in the hospital where there are high rates of hospital-based infections. Dangerous germs are often brought into hospitals by other patients who are in the hospital because they are sick, and hospital staff members are often carriers of dangerous bacteria and viruses.

Third, the absence of routine interventions like electronic fetal monitors, IVs, and medications for pain and to induce or augment labor, and the willingness of midwives to support women to labor in a range of positions—rather than insisting she hold still and lie down—means that complications are often avoided. Evidence shows that technology sets up women for more invasive practices.[5]

Fourth, the potentially dangerous overuse of obstetric interventions, such as induction and cesarean sections without adequate medical indications for them, found in most hospitals, is avoided.

Valuable Questions to Ask Yourself about Home Birth

• Are you committed to natural, medication-free childbirth?

• Do you have the support you require from your partner and family to do this?

• Have you and your midwife thoroughly evaluated your risk for complications?

• Will you feel safe and secure if you are not in or next to a hospital, knowing you can be transferred if necessary?

• How far are you from the hospital at times of usual traffic patterns?

• Are you adequately prepared to go to the hospital if the need arises?

The answers to these questions will help you determine if a home birth is right for you and your baby. Honestly, the greatest benefit of giving birth in your own home is that you don't need to do anything to prepare for it except bring in the food, beverages, and birth aids you would like to have there, such as a birth ball, a birthing stool, an inflatable tub, and so forth. In the next chapter, we'll talk about finding an excellent midwife.

Adding Your Wishes to Your Birth Plan

By now, you may feel you have decided upon the type of setting in which you'd like to have your baby. Take out your journal and, on a fresh page, write down the reasons for that selection. What features of a birth location are most important to you? As we move through this book and you absorb new information about safety and empowerment, you may revisit the step of selecting a birth location in the process of developing your final birth plan.

Some women, especially those planning out-of-hospital births at home or in a birth center, prepare two birth plans—one for a healthy birth with no complications and one for an emergency scenario in which they must be transported to the hospital. If you are leaning toward giving birth in a hospital, your next step may be to compare several hospitals in your area. Use your notes on initial wishes to guide your exploration.

As the decisions are interlinked, the next piece of crucial information we're going to look at is who you want to be with you in your chosen location as your birth attendant. What are the core issues in choosing a maternity caregiver? What are the significant differences between the medical and the midwifery models of childbirth? Does this affect your need for personal advocates and a secondary support team? Keep on reading.

Four

Selecting Your Birth Attendant

*Everything You Need to Know
About Obstetricians and Midwives*

Who should be your primary birth attendant? Answering this fundamental question goes hand in hand with your selection of a birth location and birth-planning activities. For a home birth or to give birth in an out-of-hospital birth center, your options involve the choice of a midwife. Doctors do not attend home births. So if you trust the doctor who has been serving your prepregnancy gynecological needs, and you are now committed to having this OB-GYN attend your birth, by necessity you must go to the hospital and make your future decisions based on how maternity care is handled in that setting. For hospital birth, your options would involve the choice of an obstetrician or a midwife.

When choosing your primary birth attendant, remember that anyone working in a hospital or in a birth center connected to a hospital must ascribe to the hospital's policies. Many parents have been surprised at the routines and procedures they encountered in natural birth centers that were not independent of any hospital, or "freestanding," even when nurse-midwives provided the primary maternity care in these settings.

Home-birth midwives often—not always—provide different care than in-hospital nurse-midwives. As you'll see later in the chapter, there is more than one type of midwife training.

Midwives provide continuous one-on-one care, whereas doctors typically only enter the labor setting when there's a complication or birth is imminent. Obstetricians can perform surgery, whereas midwives cannot. Yet these are not their only distinguishing features. The medical model of birth and the midwifery model of birth simply are not the same. This is partly due to the training that both types of practitioners receive and partly due to the dissimilarity of their hands-on clinical experiences within the very different contexts of hospital and freestanding birth center or home. Therefore, before you select your primary birth attendant, it is important for you to understand their philosophical distinctions. What are the pros and cons of doctors? What are the pros and cons of midwives? What questions might you ask to help you decide if you want to work with a specific practitioner?

Understanding Obstetricians

The United States and Canada are the only countries in the world where highly trained surgeons (obstetricians) supposedly attend the majority of normal, low-risk births. The American obstetrician is expected to be all things to all women, from primary-care provider for 4 million normal, healthy pregnant women every year, to specialist in complications of pregnancy and birth for 400,000 women every year, to provider of preventive gynecology, such as cancer screening and family planning, to specialist in women's diseases, and skilled surgeon. No other kind of doctor tries to maintain competence in so many areas.

Is an obstetrician truly able to do six hours of painstaking gynecological surgery on a woman with extensive cancer, and then rush to the office and do the best job of patiently counseling a healthy pregnant woman about her sex life? Not likely.

Because obstetricians are surgeons, they often turn birth into a surgical procedure. Proof of this is that the birthing woman is treated as though she is a surgical patient by putting her on her back in a bed, which is really a modified surgical table, often with her legs up in surgical stirrups. As we discussed earlier, scientifically, this is the worst of all possible positions for the woman giving birth, as in this position the baby's head compresses the woman's main blood vessel supplying the womb and the baby. If the woman is in a vertical position (sitting, squatting, or standing), more blood and oxygen goes to the baby, the woman's bony pelvis opens wider to let the baby out, and she gives birth "downhill" instead of "uphill" against gravity.

A good way of finding out whether or not an individual doctor or hospital is practicing modern maternity care is simple: Just ask what position women are put in during birth. If they are still putting women on their backs during birth, they are viewing birth as a surgical procedure.

Statistics show that approximately 5 to 10 percent of births involve serious medical complications that are best managed with a medical and surgical approach.[1] Obstetricians are essential in such cases. But the obstetricians' plate is full to overflowing in America, and there is no way they can do it all. Of all the tasks they try to accomplish, the one that by far takes the most time is childbirth, which on average lasts twelve hours and can happen night or day, seven days a week.

Official statistics report that doctors are the primary birth attendants in more than 90 percent of births. In reality, for most hospital births, the real birth attendant is the labor-and-delivery nurse. After completing basic nursing training, this professional nurse typically receives an additional six weeks of training in labor-and-delivery nursing. In the maternity ward, as she is usually responsible for simultaneously monitoring several women in labor, she can rarely provide an individual woman with continuous one-on-one care. Eight-hour shift changes among the staff also means there is no possibility for continuous monitoring by the same nurse during a woman's entire labor.

Data prove that unfragmented care from the same birth attendant correlates with shorter labor, less pain, fewer complications, and better outcomes.[2] Unfortunately, the only women likely to get this safest, most effective type of care during labor and birth are the less than 10 percent who have chosen to be attended by a midwife, rather than an obstetrician and his or her hospital's team of labor-and-delivery nurses.

As someone interested in having a safe and empowering woman-centered birth, what guideposts can help you to evaluate an obstetrician's quality? Check the doctor's credentials and ask about rates of intervention in labor with drugs, technology, and surgery. Good doctors are able to provide most of their intervention rates, such as for cesarean sections, off the top of their heads. It isn't necessary that you like and befriend your doctor; however, you should have the sense that your doctor respects you and is placing your needs above his or her own. A doctor should have time enough to discuss all of your concerns about your labor, return your phone calls in a timely manner, be open to getting a second opinion, and show overt respect for midwives, nurses, and other staff.

If you ask a doctor, "What do you think?" and you receive a condescending or sarcastic response, it should be a red light. Use the valuable questions on pages 66–67, for more guidance in ascertaining whether or not you are comfortable with a specific doctor.

Problems with the Surgical Mind-set

Having an obstetric surgeon attend a healthy birth is like having a pediatric surgeon baby-sit a healthy two-year-old. Both are going to be tempted to apply medical solutions to everyday situations, such as using drugs to stimulate normal labor or narcotics to put a fussy toddler to sleep. Unfortunately, using highly trained surgeons to handle normal life experiences, such as childbirth, increases unnecessary and risky interventions, decreases women's satisfaction, and wastes huge amounts of money.

A major problem arising from the obstetric near-monopoly over childbirth in America is the extreme medicalization of normal pregnancy and birth. To see the flaw in this approach, it's instructive to look at the history of obstetrics and what has happened when doctors have managed normal birth like it was a medical event. In the eighteenth and nineteenth centuries, there was an epidemic of deaths of women during childbirth—childbed fever. This epidemic was occurring in women who had chosen to go to the hospital to give birth, and it was not occurring in women who stayed home to give birth assisted by a midwife. In 1795, a Scottish scientist by the name of Alexander Gordon proved it was the result of doctors who, after examining sick patients, then went from one laboring woman to another without washing their hands. They were transferring the deadly bacteria that always reside in hospitals with sick people in them to these women and killing them. In 1843, Oliver Wendell Holmes, one of the most famous of American medical men and a professor at Harvard, published an essay agreeing with Gordon, and in 1847, Ignaz Philipp Semmelweis in Vienna brought about a 6 percent drop in mortality in women at his maternity hospital simply by requiring hand washing by staff.

Gordon's work was ignored, Holmes's essay was ignored, and poor Semmelweis lost his job and was driven out of Vienna. All their good information was greeted with hostility by obstetricians, who refused to believe the terrible epidemic of deaths of women giving birth could be their fault. And it was not until the 1880s, ninety years after the true cause and way to stop the epidemic of deaths had been determined, and not until many thousands of women had died needlessly, that hospitals and governments made regulations forcing doctors to wash their hands, leading to the abrupt end of the deadly epidemic.

Medicalization of normal pregnancy and birth continued in the twentieth century. The 1930s saw routine X-raying of the woman's pelvis during pregnancy, before research proved that it caused cancer in the baby. The 1950s saw widespread use of the drug diethylstilbestrol (DES) during pregnancy, before research proved it caused defects in the baby's reproductive organs. The 1970s saw widespread use of the drug thalidomide during pregnancy, before research proved it caused deformities of the arms and legs in babies. The 1990s saw yet another example of extreme medicalization of normal birth by obstetricians resulting in doctor-caused adverse outcomes: widespread use of the drug Cytotec for labor induction, before research proved it markedly increased the risk of rupture of the uterus in a woman with a previous cesarean section, thus causing women and babies to die.

Although the consensus wave of the future in medical practice is practice based on the best scientific evidence, many doctors still believe that much of the time what to do for a patient is a judgment call based on past experience. This allows them to insist that unless you were there at the time and unless you have had as much clinical experience as they have, you can't criticize what they did. And this position goes a step further: Neither can you evaluate their performance based on data on groups of patients (cesarean-section rates for a given hospital, for example), since it's necessary to consider all aspects of each individual case and, in the final analysis, use clinical judgment. Clinical judgment, then, is an attempt by the clinicians to reject what the scientific evidence says they should be doing. Any scientist who tries to evaluate the actions of obstetricians frequently hears these sorts of arguments.

Subtle Factors That Influence Doctors to Intervene in the Birth Process

Rarely during prenatal visits do obstetricians tell women the truth about their impending absence during labor, which sadly—and rightfully—leaves women feeling neglected and deserted when they come to the hospital in labor. Yet, in order to attract women to their practices, doctors tell women: "Come to me, with all my expertise, and come to my hospital, with all its incredible technology, and you will have a perfect birth and beautiful baby." Women are not always informed that interventions have risks.

Since obstetricians have been specially trained to manage the few cases of truly high-risk birth—situations where things can and do go wrong—obstetricians often end up fearing the birth process. Imagine an auto mechanic who only sees Fords that have broken down and been brought to him for repairs. He ends up thinking that all Fords are in imminent danger of breaking down, while forgetting that he never sees the Fords on the road that are running fine. Likewise, a pervasive sense that "trouble is imminent" leads some obstetricians to jump in way too early with interventions.

Another subtle underlying factor that drives some obstetricians to promote radical, invasive interventions is their fundamental belief in machines and fundamental lack of belief in women and their bodies. Most obstetricians routinely use electronic fetal heart monitors in spite of clear scientific evidence, and the recommendations of the ACOG, that a good old stethoscope is just as reliable and has better results.[3] When the method of estimating the length of pregnancy using ultrasound technology came along, obstetricians immediately dropped the tried-and-true method of asking women about their last menstrual cycles. Even to this day, estimating the length of pregnancy with ultrasound is not very accurate, as the true length of gestation can vary by as much as two weeks on either side of the due date given by the ultrasound—short or long. Women's menstrual dates remain just as reliable a way to estimate what their due dates will be. But obstetricians will generally ask for ultrasound dating and trust that result, rather than trust a woman's knowledge about her body.

Because the vast majority of obstetricians have only experienced hospital-based, medical births, they cannot truly see the profound effect their interventions have on the process.[4] By separating a woman from her own environment and surrounding her with strange people using strange machines that do strange things to her, her state of mind and body are so altered that her way of carrying through this intimate act of giving birth must also be altered. The entire modern, published literature in obstetrics is based on observations of "medicalized" birth. It is not possible for obstetricians to know what births would have been like without these manipulations, as they have not personally experienced natural birth.

How Are Doctors Trained?

For the most part, obstetricians are hardworking and want the best for the women they serve. They're caring people. But years of isolation in the obstetric world can leave them mired in and blinded by the point of view of the obstetric establishment. Although they don't sit down and consciously decide on it, most obstetricians nonetheless internalize a set of assumptions during their training and careers, and one of the most potent is that maternity care should be seen in obstetricians' terms, rather than women's terms.

Organized obstetrics has the characteristics of a tribe. First is a long period of preparation that begins with four undergraduate years at college. Then, when students are accepted at medical school they begin their next four years of study with a rite of passage: Each is handed a white coat, the symbol of their new status. Medical school is full of lessons on status and hierarchy. During the four years in medical school, the education is not only medical but also social. They are taught how to behave as doctors and think as doctors. Eight years of undergraduate and medical school are followed by a year of internship and then three or four years of specialty training in obstetrics and gynecology. It's no accident that those in specialty training are called "residents," as their duties demand that, for all practical purposes, they reside at the hospital. They are living in a more and more narrow, closed world surrounded by "tribal elders."

Finally, obstetricians go through examinations for board certification. Their process of preparation, which takes so long and is so intense, results in strong feelings of pride in and loyalty to the tribe and to the obstetrical establishment. Because of the long educational purgatory, it also can result in feelings of entitlement and arrogance.

Now the young obstetrician enters the insular world of obstetrics. He or she frequently goes to hospital "obstetric grand rounds," where cases are discussed, occasionally to local meetings of the obstetric society or regional meetings of the ACOG, and perhaps to national ACOG meetings. And from time to time the obstetrician will, with financial help from a pharmaceutical company, go on a cruise or to a ski resort for obstetric conferences, where a few hours are devoted each day to lectures. In every one of these meetings, the obstetrician only hears current obstetric dogma. Yet, when all is said and done, many obstetricians come out of all this with a caring attitude and a genuine wish to help women—and these are the ones you are looking for, of course.

Never once during obstetrical training are doctors required to sit with a woman throughout her entire labor and birth. As a result, obstetricians have little experience with normal, healthy births, but a whole lot of experience with those few births where serious complications occur. At those times, their training and take-charge mind-set are valuable.

The Important Role of Labor-and-Delivery Nurses

The task of the labor-and-delivery nurse is thankless and often impossible: to try to closely monitor several women in labor at once. The fact that defines and limits these nurses is that they have very little autonomy and can do almost nothing that goes beyond routine nursing care without doctors' orders. If problems develop, the labor-and-delivery nurse has no authority to act except to try to find the doctor. Additionally, she (or occasionally he) must try to judge the moment of birth accurately. If she calls the doctor too soon, she wastes the doctor's time. If she calls the doctor too late, the doctor misses the birth. The doctor is supposed to show up to catch the baby at the end of labor.

Only the United States and Canada have this fragmented system for managing labor and birth, and the Canadians are rapidly training midwives to replace obstetricians for normal births. In other highly developed countries, literally in more than 75 percent of pregnancies, it is a midwife who provides all prenatal care, admits the woman in labor to the hospital, attends the labor, and is the primary attendant at the hospital birth. In many countries, after giving birth a woman goes home from the hospital never having laid eyes on a doctor.

If you give birth in a hospital, the hospital's labor-and-delivery nurses will actually be your primary caregivers whenever a doctor isn't present, which is most of the time. Doctors usually aren't present for the majority of their patients' labors. In some instances, the doula and nurses will simultaneously care for you, with the nurse handling clinical matters. But you won't ever have a choice of nurses in a hospital, as they are staff members assigned by a head nurse to care for you and other laboring women, and they must rotate according to their shift schedules.

A good labor-and-delivery nurse is a wonderful ally to a woman in labor. She can be an important source of information in the informed consent and refusal process and help the birthing woman identify natural alternatives to drugs and high-tech procedures. The labor-and-delivery nurse knows what to anticipate during childbirth, and she can encourage a woman to keep going and trust her body when the woman feels anxious. If something goes wrong, she can support the mother emotionally by reassuring her that she did her best. When the baby has been born, the labor-and-delivery nurse can create an atmosphere for the mother to bond with her newborn.

A labor-and-delivery nurse can also be an impediment to a woman's birth plan. As the nurses frequently set the tone in the maternity ward, a problematic nurse can often serve as an invasive—perhaps even hostile—presence in the labor room and may try to override the laboring woman. Unfortunately, if you are subjected to such treatment, you'll need to stand up for yourself. You can protect yourself by bringing an advocate—your spouse or a doula—who can run interference for you. You can also go up the chain of command and complain to the nursing supervisor. That should correct the problem.

You are not required to be nice to everyone around you when you're in labor. Well-trained nurses are capable of handling irritable or needy birthing women. They have seen it all and most won't take your behavior personally. Moaning and complaining is allowable. You are the center of the experience when you're in labor. Queen for a day.

In most cases, though, labor-and-delivery nurses are in an advantageous position to remind doctors and other staff members what a woman's birth plan requests. By dropping a word in edgewise as a subtle reminder to doctors, they can buy a woman time before invasive procedures get forcefully suggested to her. Nurses can run interference with other personnel to create a safe environment and halt unwanted measures from being taken in the nick of time. As much as the hospital allows, they can be advocates for safer, evidence-based practices.

Understanding Midwives

A few years ago, during a panel discussion on a TV talk show, a practicing obstetrician said: "Midwives are obstetrician's assistants." As a fellow panelist, I tried to correct his misperception: Having obstetricians supervise midwives is like having Coca-Cola supervise Pepsi. They are different, yes, but equal. Through no fault of our own, Americans have little understanding of midwifery. In the early twentieth century, a medical witch-hunt against midwives in the United States resulted in their elimination as a legitimate healthcare profession. As a consequence, most of us usually have no personal experience with midwives and, in addition, have received considerable misinformation about midwifery.

A Brief History of Midwifery

Midwives have always been with us. They are the women in the community to whom other women can turn for support with their problems. "Midwife" is Old English for "with woman." The French word for midwife, *sage femme* (wise woman), goes back thousands of years, as does the Danish word for midwife, *jordmor* (earth mother), and the Icelandic word for midwife, *ljosmodir* (mother of light). It is extremely rare to find a male midwife, so the pronoun "she" will be used to describe midwives in this book.

Hippocrates started a midwifery-training program in Greece in the fifth century B.C. Phaenarete, mother of Socrates, was a midwife. In the Bible, the book of Exodus recognizes the strength and independence of midwives who defied the pharaoh's command to kill all sons born to Hebrew women. Before America was "discovered," the first law to regulate European midwifery was passed in Germany in 1452. Since then, and without interruption to the present time, every little girl in Europe grows up with the understanding that if she ever has a baby, she will have a midwife assist her.

As Europeans migrated to the New World, midwives were among

them. In the mid-1600s, the king of France commissioned midwives working in New France (now Canada) and the British government paid for the services of midwives in the New World. Midwives were a valued part of the developing healthcare system, participating in the teaching of medical students in at least one university in the mid-1880s. As the number of physicians increased in America, they attempted to monopolize healthcare through medical practice acts. By the end of the nineteenth century midwives were being accused of witchcraft and tried in court, and so began to disappear. Nurses supported the medical domination of maternity care. An attempt to open a school of midwifery in Massachusetts in 1910 was defeated by opposition from both nurses and physicians.

Yet, throughout history every attempt at stamping out midwifery has failed. There will always be women who want to be midwives and women who want midwives at the birth of their children. So when officially sanctioned midwifery disappeared in America, many midwives simply went underground. "Granny midwives" continued to serve poor women. And in Appalachia, where there were no doctors, the government formed the "Frontier Nursing Service" to bring healthcare to this remote area. Soon these nurses were catching babies, creating a new profession, the nurse-midwife, in America.

Nurse-midwifery grew slowly but surely, and midwives who did not want to train first as nurses developed direct-entry midwifery, which also steadily grew in numbers and recognition. A direct-entry midwife is a midwife who is trained in the profession of midwifery without previous training in nursing. Special schools of midwifery exist for this type of midwife and there are national standardized examinations for accreditation. By the year 2000, every state was licensing nurse-midwives, and more than half of the states were licensing direct-entry midwives, with new states being added to the list every year. At present, the U.S. federal government recognizes the professional training for both types of midwives and approves of their national examinations.

Recent U.S. government–sponsored research proves that midwives are actually safer than obstetricians for the 80-plus percent of births that have no serious medical complications no matter where they work, whether in or out of hospitals.[5] That's because the care they provide tends to be more "mother friendly," with more continuous, one-on-one care than the care provided in the average hospital setting by doctors and the teams of labor-and-delivery nurses that assist them. Midwives have had more training and more experience in normal birth than either obstetricians or labor-and-delivery nurses. And because midwives have more experience with normal birth, understand variations of normal better, and are not constantly anxious that something may go wrong, they have far lower rates of interventions—induction, episiotomy, forceps and vacuum extraction, cesarean section—when compared with doctors who also are attending low-risk births. American midwifery is a rapidly expanding field. Many of the largest HMOs in the country now employ more midwives than obstetricians, and midwives attend most of the births under some of the HMOs' auspices.

What Is a Midwife?

With the current renaissance of midwifery, a century of ignorance and confusion about midwifery must be overcome. Myths surround midwives, implying that midwives are "hippies," "religious zealots," or "witches with magical potions." Another belief is that midwifery is "second-class obstetrics for those who can't get an obstetrician." None of these myths and misconceptions is true. The practice of midwifery is very different from the practice of nursing and medicine.

Midwifery is primary care for women. While often limited to maternity care, it may include other aspects of women's reproductive health, such as family planning and reproductive tract infections. A midwife is analogous to a family physician in providing primary care and referring to specialist care as needed. A midwife transferring a laboring woman to an obstetrician when complications arise that may require surgery is analogous to a family physician referring a patient with blocked arteries to a cardiologist.

Midwives insist that pregnancy is not an illness. They know what can go wrong, how to identify problems early, and to cooperate with doctors in managing complications. They also know that while pursuing medical aspects of pregnancy is essential, it is not enough. They are trained to go beyond medical care and support the pregnant woman to achieve her goals for herself and her baby. Midwives use low-tech assistance, such as the skilled use of their hands, and understand the importance of preserving normalcy in childbirth. Midwives believe in women's bodies and their capacity to reproduce with little or no intervention in most cases. The key elements in the midwifery model are normality, facilitation of natural processes with the minimal amount of evidence-based interventions, and the empowerment of the woman.

An important difference between low-risk births attended by midwives and obstetricians is the emotional quality of the care given. Many surveys have shown a far higher level of satisfaction with a woman's birth experience if a midwife rather than an obstetrician attends childbirth. This is not hard to understand. If you have selected a midwife as your birth attendant, she will be with you from the beginning of labor until some time after the birth is completed. An obstetrician will pop in on you from time to time, while in between, you will be seen intermittently by a nurse. Since the average length of labor is twelve hours, and nurses change shifts every eight hours, it is very likely that you will be faced with not one, but two different strangers popping into your hospital room from time to time to check on you in the absence of your doctor.

Besides being there all the time and giving the woman as much control as is possible given the situation, midwifery has other attributes that offer a level of satisfaction not possible with obstetric care. Whenever the doctor runs a test or gives a treatment to a laboring woman, it can be an unspoken vote of no confidence in her body. While the occasional test is a good idea, often they only serve to reassure fearful doctors.

As the midwife continuously uses every means possible to demonstrate her belief in the ability of the woman's body to give birth successfully, the woman herself begins to believe in her abilities. The result can be an incredibly empowering birthing experience. Since this same woman is now faced with the daunting task of spending the next twenty years raising her child, believing in herself and her abilities is vital to her mothering skills.

How Are Midwives Trained?

For 100 years, the apprenticeship model has been the foundation of the medical training of physicians. Direct-entry midwifery training uses the apprenticeship model as well. A midwife learns about prenatal care and catching babies under the supervision of a fully qualified mentor, and after documenting the minimum experience required, takes a set of standard examinations to test her understanding of a body of knowledge gained through independent study. This training is officially approved by the U.S. Department of Education.

The renaissance the past two decades of direct-entry midwifery in the United States is based on the development of the North American Registry of Midwives (NARM) standardized national examination and the Certified Professional Midwife (CPM) process. Educators view the NARM examination and CPM process as exemplary programs, as they utilize the apprenticeship and distant-learning approaches, both of which are seen as progressive steps in the education of all healthcare professionals. The World Health Organization definition of a midwife neither contains the words "nurse," "obstetrician," or "supervision," nor does it specify the length or type of education the midwife must have or any academic degrees she must hold. In states that have approved and licensed direct-entry midwives, the CPM meets the official definition of a midwife.

The standardization and testing of the NARM examination has been more thorough than nearly any other medical or nursing examination. There can be no doubt that a midwife who has passed the NARM examination and is a CPM is competent to carry out all necessary procedures during birth, including administering oxygen, giving drugs, performing competent neonatal resuscitation, and so forth. This is because the apprenticeship process includes both formal and informal instruction in every basic scientific and clinical subject necessary for the practice of competent midwifery.

In recent years, more than half of the states have passed legislation that legalizes direct-entry midwives and planned out-of-hospital birth. In approximately sixteen of these states, the legislation uses the NARM examination and CPM certification. Sometimes medical and obstetrical societies have testified against the legislation, claiming there's a lack of safety in home birth, but without any scientific data to back up such claims. After careful consideration of the scientific evidence, every one of the legislatures has found direct-entry midwives and planned out-of-hospital births to be a safe option for their citizens.

Many obstetricians continue to use what they consider to be the pejorative label of "lay midwives" when describing these women. Ironically, such midwives aren't allowed to take a standardized national examination until they have attended at least fifty births, while a nurse need not document *any* experience as a birth attendant before being assigned to monitor women in labor, and many doctors finish medical school having attended *one or two* births—if they are lucky. Nurse-midwives go through rigorous four-year university training programs that combine clinical work and course work, and which qualify them at the end to give primary healthcare to women. Upon satisfactory completion of the program, the student sits for examination by the American Midwifery Certification Board. The good news is that nurse-midwives mainly provide midwifery care to women giving birth in hospitals—where most childbirth takes place in America—either as independent practitioners or as members of an obstetric group. The bad news is that hospital-based nurse-midwives must struggle daily to practice real midwifery and not become "medwives" who do obstetricians' biddings and accept the medical model of birth.

Differences Among Midwives

Perhaps the biggest source of confusion for the consumer of maternity services is to understand the difference between midwives who work at in-hospital birth centers and midwives who work at out-of-hospital birth centers. In-hospital birth centers and out-of-hospital birth centers function according to distinct models of care: the medical model and the midwifery model. Within an in-hospital birth center—a facility that's closely affiliated with a hospital—most likely one or more of the midwives on the staff would attend you, rotating in shifts as happens in a hospital birth. Nurses are doctors' assistants by both training and practice, and are literally given "doctor's orders." They are not allowed to do more than a few basic patient-care practices without first consulting a doctor. The patient belongs to a given doctor, who is responsible for the overall care of that person. Midwives, on the other hand, are not doctors' assistants. They are independent professionals with expertise in normal, or low-risk, birth. They don't usually take "doctor's orders," but rather collaborate with doctors in mutually deciding what the care will be.

With home-birth midwives, it is clear that the birthing woman is in control of her labor and makes final decisions regarding what will happen. This is not always easy for midwives working in hospital settings to promise, as they are subject to hospital policy, which may include rules about mandatory IVs, electronic monitoring, withholding food and beverages, and imposed time limits on the first and second stages of labor.

While a hospital-based midwife or a midwife who transfers her client to a hospital for complications may argue on behalf of her client against hospital rules, the reality is that I have never seen a hospital where the patient or midwife is truly in control.

If you want a midwife to provide your primary maternity care, find one who has as much autonomy as possible in her practice. That may mean avoiding in-hospital birth centers. If you are considering having a particular obstetrician provide your primary maternity care, a good way to measure that doctor's openness and attitude toward you and women in general is to inquire what his or her opinion is of midwifery.

It's much easier for obstetricians to control nurse-midwives since most nurse-midwives work in obstetricians' offices and hospitals and take orders from obstetricians. In the past, accommodation was a central strategy of nurse-midwives, trying to live in the doctor's world and survive.

Choosing the Right Maternity Care Provider for You

Talk to the midwives and doctors available to you. Interview them at length, watching to see if they get restless or uncomfortable. Tell them that giving birth is one of the most important events in your life and you will go to whatever lengths to have it done right. Examine their faces closely as you tell them that you want an empowering birth. Are they condescending and do they seem to resent your questions? Or do they encourage you to take responsibility for your own pregnancy and birth? Don't be afraid to change care providers if after a few visits you don't like how one is caring (or not caring) for you.

Midwives use low-tech assistance, such as the skilled use of their hands, and understand the importance of preserving normalcy in childbirth. They have good hands and know how to sit on them. Obstetricians in general use high-tech assistance and focus on the pursuit of abnormality. Every technology and procedure comes with risks. You have to decide for yourself the risks you are willing to assume during labor.

Sheryl Rivett, activist and mother of four children born at home, conducted a research study, *Mothers and Midwives,* for which she gathered numerous stories of women's midwifery experiences. In an interview, she told me that most of the stories she heard were incredibly positive and life affirming. Only a few were negative. Of course, any caregiver can have serious personal problems, and you need to be on the alert for them. Whether they are a midwife, a doctor, a doula, a nurse, or anesthesiologist, they need to be carefully evaluated.

Just always remember, every potential caregiver you consider is a human first and a caregiver second. That is as true for obstetricians as it is for midwives.

Finding a Good Obstetrician

When deciding on your primary maternity-care provider, it is important to ask the obstetrician about his or her practices.

- May I phone you when labor starts to get advice on when to come to the hospital and if I am permitted to stay at home during part of the first stage of labor?

- How often can I expect to see you during labor?

- How likely is it that you'll be present when I give birth?

- If not, who will be there instead? Can I meet them?

- Can I meet your partner (partners)?

- What prenatal tests do you use?

- Do you prefer to put a woman on her back during birth? (See chapter 5.)

- Can I labor in any position I want, including vertical positions during the second stage? And, what equipment do you have to make this possible (for example, birth ball, birth stools, ceiling rope, and so on)—or can I bring my own props with me?

- How often do you do episiotomy? (See chapter 8.)

- What percent of your clients are induced? (See chapter 6.)

- What percent of your clients are augmented? (See chapter 6.)

- What percent of your clients have forceps or vacuum extraction? (See chapter 5.)

- What percent of your clients have cesarean section? (See chapter 8.)

- How many women in your practice give birth without pharmacological pain relief? (See chapter 7.)

- Is electronic fetal monitoring routine with all births? And, can my baby's heart be monitored with a fetoscope rather than electronically? (See chapter 5.)

- Can my baby's heart be intermittently, rather than continuously, monitored?

- Can I eat and drink in labor?

- Can I labor without receiving IV fluids? (See chapter 5.)

- Can I walk around and move freely in labor?

- Is there a time limit for labor? How long can I push?

- [If female and a mother] May I ask if you have ever given birth vaginally?

- [If male and a father] May I ask if your children were born vaginally?

- Will you wait to cut the umbilical cord until it stops pulsating?

- Can you put the baby on my chest (skin-to-skin contact) after birth and have the newborn exam done there?

- Can I breastfeed in the first half hour after birth?

- If I write a birth plan, will you honor it? In your absence, will your partners and staff honor it?

If the doctor resists giving you the data or doesn't know his or her intervention rates, watch out. Beware of any tendency to patronize you and suggest that you cannot possibly understand technical information about childbirth. Review the "mother-friendly" maternity-care guidelines in chapter 1 to see statistically appropriate intervention rates. If the doctor's practice deviates from these, ask, "Why?" Watch out for excuses, such as: "I have lots of high-risk patients."

Finding a Good Midwife

First, you need to determine the legal status of midwives in your state. Contact state midwifery associations or the midwives' organization listed in the Resources section of this book. Remember that CPMs and certified nurse-midwives (CNMs) should practice the midwifery model of care. CPMs are mostly direct-entry midwives who've met the qualifications for the CPM credential. Other direct-entry midwives may have state qualifications without receiving outside certification. CNMs are educated in both nursing and midwifery and rarely assist home births. Take the names of any midwives you receive by referral and check their credentials. Also interview them.

If you opt for giving birth in an out-of-hospital birth center, you'll meet a team of midwives who back one another up. Sit down with them and ask questions, too. What you may discover is that, unlike home-birth midwives who can spend up to an hour, they only spend fifteen minutes or so with you during prenatal visits.

Some CPMs and CNMs do *not* closely follow the midwifery model of care, just as not all doctors closely follow the medical model. There's a range of approaches and degrees of intervention. So it's important to ask plenty of questions. In selecting a midwife, as acclaimed midwife and author Ina May Gaskin pointed out in a 2005 interview with me, "Use your common sense. If a practitioner is inebriated or rude when you meet her, this is evidently not someone you want attending you during childbirth." Midwives are human beings, and you may or may not get along well with every one of them. "Be a smart shopper."

Valuable Questions for Midwives

Ask your candidate midwives these questions, and any others that come to mind.

• How, when, and where did you receive your midwifery education?

• Are you certified or licensed?

- What physician collaboration or backup do you have?

- Do you have privileges in a hospital? (Meaning, can she assist you there herself?)

- Do you have a good working relationship with obstetricians in the hospital?

- Do you maintain statistics from your practice? May I see them?

- Do you work with a partner (partners)? If so, what are her (their) qualifications?

- What prenatal tests do you use?

- How many women are due within a month of my due date?

- What is your plan if someone else is in labor when I am?

- Do you use pharmaceutical products to induce or augment labor?

- Do you use herbs to induce or augment labor?

- Do you carry an oxygen tank to births?

- What methods do you suggest to alleviate labor pain?

- What laboring positions are recommended?

- Is your certification in neonatal resuscitation up to date?

- To what hospital do you transport if it becomes necessary? Will you come with me if there is a need for cesarean section?

- How long will you stay with me after my baby is born?

- How often will you make postpartum visits?

- Do you participate in regular peer review?

- If I write a birth plan, will you honor it? In your absence, will your partners honor it?

Adding Your Wishes to Your Birth Plan

Based on the discussions in this chapter, I am sure you can see clearly how doctors and midwives approach childbirth from different, yet complementary perspectives. You may have developed a preference already for one type of maternity care. If you have opted to labor at home or in a birth center, you are now engaged in a process of locating and interviewing midwives to find the right match for you. If you have opted for a hospital birth, you are now engaged in selecting an appropriate doctor or nurse-midwife under whose care you feel comfortable laboring. Keep notes in your journal of what is said during meetings with maternity-care providers and of your personal discoveries.

If you were under the care of an OB-GYN prior to pregnancy and you would like to maintain that relationship throughout childbirth, this is the time to sit down and have a preliminary chat about your wishes, specifically your emerging vision of an ideal labor. Now that your needs have changed, you and your past caregiver may or may not mesh as well as you once did. Or you may find that your connection deepens and trust grows. Again, keep a record of what is said and any new questions that arise. You'll be put on a schedule of regular appointments, so there will be many chances to dialogue.

Having chosen your primary healthcare provider, you are now ready to explore the kinds of interventions most likely to be suggested to you or to be required by that kind of provider during labor and birth. What are the ramifications of the initial decisions you made about birth location and birth attendant? In the next chapter, we'll look at ways to prepare ahead of time to handle commonly used birth technology and consider some of the alternatives to these devices.

Five

Ensuring the Appropriate Use of Birth Technology

Electronic Fetal Monitors, IVs, Forceps, and Vacuum Extractors

Before the birth of her son, Natalie had prepared for a home water birth. Labor began a few days after the due date and at first everything went according to the plan. At 10 A.M., the midwife arrived. Natalie's pains were getting stronger and her husband, Andrew, microwaved an herbal heat wrap and put it on her back. She leaned forward over a chair and he massaged her. The pool was set up. Natalie moved around freely. She would lie in bed, get up, walk around, and go to the toilet. By 1:30 P.M., she was six centimeters dilated. The midwife guessed the baby would come soon. At 3 P.M. Natalie was fully dilated and started pushing. She and her husband were given a lot of privacy. Even the midwife and her assistant left the room at one point to take a break and drink a smoothie. The couple kissed.

Natalie reports, "This was the perfect experience. Even though I was in pain, it was a pain I knew I could deal with. Even the pushing was gratifying. I actually enjoyed it because I kept thinking of the result: We were going to have a baby." Natalie's labor was heroic. She was pushing on the bed and the midwife tried to find her a good position to push the baby down and out. They could see the top of the baby's head and thought he was coming. But he wasn't moving. So Natalie started doing "sumo-wrestler" squats on the floor. She did about five while Andrew held her up. Then she got back on the bed, shifted onto her hands and knees, and tried pushing like that. Then she did more squats. Then she went back on the toilet. The midwife kept checking heart tones to see if the baby was in distress. They could find his heartbeat and he was OK.

After two hours of pushing, the midwives left the room. Natalie sensed that her pushing needed to be more focused and concentrated. The baby needed to come out. She did sumo-wrestler squats, lifting one leg or the other. It was intense and painful to do when she was in a contraction. Plus it was exhausting. Then the midwife came back and said, "If the baby doesn't come in half an hour, we'll have to go to the hospital." They had already alerted everyone else in the house that Natalie would need to go; yet they continued to support her to try to give birth naturally. They didn't want her to lose focus. Natalie wasn't anxious. But she was more and more exhausted.

"We have to go," the midwife finally said. Then it was a mad rush. Natalie, who was naked, put on a robe, walked to the car, and sat in the front seat. It was painful. She had to breathe through strong contractions and couldn't push in the car. They drove over speed bumps and tiny road bumps on the five-minute trip to the hospital. She couldn't sit in the wheelchair they offered her in the emergency room. She walked to the elevator.

In the maternity ward, Natalie was put in a room and the nurses immediately began hooking up electronic monitors and rushing around her. She was relieved, because she was tired. She knew that if anything happened they could handle it. Everything she hadn't wanted started happening and she had to surrender to it. Natalie had read to be flexible about the birth outcome, so she tried to look at the process from a spiritual point of view. For whatever reason, the baby needed this experience even if it made her sad that her expectations weren't being met.

She says, "The nurses were so incredible. I have huge respect for the nursing profession. They were like goddesses to me. This one nurse, Christine, said, 'We can see his head. You can have this baby naturally.'

She started coaching me with the pushing. She was focused and good. It was exactly what I needed. I was still convinced I could do it naturally."

The medical team explained interventions to Natalie before they did them and she asked questions. They had put a monitor on her belly. A doctor visited her to explain that an epidural might help her relax so she could still have the baby vaginally. He was a fantastic guy, gentle and sweet. Natalie had an epidural, and then a catheter was put in. They took blood and administered tests. She kept pushing.

Then, even though she was preregistered, she had to sign consent forms. An epidural is invasive and required special consent. Because she was still feeling pain, they gave her another dose. Then everything went numb and she couldn't feel the pushing. She could only see contractions on the monitor.

The staff put an electrode on the top of his head, an internal fetal monitor. Then they said, "We're going to use forceps. We thought suction originally, but his head is swollen from being squeezed." They reassured Natalie as best they could. The midwife stayed with her the whole time, only moving into the background to let the doctors and nurses do what they had to do.

Ultimately, they had to perform a cesarean section. As Natalie says, "By then I had surrendered. As much as I believe in all-natural birth, there was relief. I wanted my baby out and I wanted him to be born safely." They wheeled her to the operating room.

Three weeks later, Natalie visited the surgeon for a checkup. "I have to ask," she told him, "did I push right? What else could I have done?" He reassured her, "There was nothing else. You did those squats and you went way beyond what was expected." Natalie had broken her tailbone when she was eleven and that might have been part of the problem. "Your baby was big. He weighed nine pounds with a head fourteen inches around. If you'd had a baby under seven pounds, you might have been able to deliver vaginally."

In Natalie's case, the technological interventions she had were necessary and her attendants beautifully supported her, first at home and then in the hospital, to give birth according to her birth plan. As a result, she gave birth to a healthy baby boy whom she treasures. She knows that extra steps needed to be taken to ensure this positive outcome. But many women, unlike Natalie, are unnecessarily subjected to invasive technology.

So how can you determine whether or not you want a particular technology or intervention to be used during your child's birth? And what factors should be considered when technological interventions are being offered? This chapter will explore the pros and cons of common interventions (both high-tech and low-tech), including IVs, fetal monitors, forceps, and vacuum extractors, and more.

When Is Birth Technology Warranted?

Midwives, especially in home-birth settings, rely on birth technology that is much less invasive than the technology so often used by midwives and doctors in hospital-birth settings. In fact, one of the main reasons a woman would be working with a midwife, besides the desire to have a home birth, is her desire to have a natural or low-tech experience. So, although a midwife uses listening devices and can offer a woman an IV if necessary, the issue of birth technology largely applies to hospital births under the care of physicians.

The stated goal of every obstetric textbook is to teach doctors to provide their patients with evidence-based medicine. Unfortunately, in many cases, there is a gap between what most doctors and hospitals do and what science says they should be doing—and the gap lies in the direction of doctors doing too much, rather than too little.[1]

Intervening in childbirth when it's not necessary is dangerous, as the need for interventions can cascade. For instance, using an epidural may slow down the progress of labor and thus result in the need for another intervention. Or a false reading from an electronic fetal monitor (EFM) may alarm birth attendants and trigger them to interfere. Many obstetricians are concerned about closing the gap between practice and science, but we have a long way to go. Woman-centered childbirth uses less technology and is more scientific. Remember not to confuse science with machines.

After World War II, a belief in the power of machines to solve every kind of problem developed in our culture. Many interventions, including ultrasound and EFM, came into widespread use without adequate scientific evaluation. We had nuclear weapons and could send a rocket to the moon. Routine childbirth was moved to hospitals and the stampede to provide high-tech birth for everyone gained momentum.

The most important reason for the dramatic decreases in the mortality of birthing women and babies in the last 100 years has not been advances in medical care or machines, but rather improvements in social and economic conditions, including better nutrition, better housing, and family planning, all of which enabled women to avoid having too many babies, and having them too early or too late in life. It was not high-tech medical and surgical interventions, such as EFM and ultrasound, but basic medical advances, such as the discovery of antibiotics to cure infections and the ability to give safe blood transfusions, that caused an improvement in birth outcomes, as did improved hygiene two hundred years ago when doctors substantially reduced the spread of "childbed fever" simply by washing their hands between patients.

Use the following information to educate yourself about the various kinds of birth technology you may be offered and to help you evaluate your feelings about them when it comes to developing a birth plan. Let's start with the most obvious common practice.

When Is Wearing Gowns and Masks Necessary?

Wearing gowns and masks in the average labor and delivery room is pure Hollywood—doctors and nurses playacting "doctors and nurses." This practice has been repeatedly proven to have no value in childbirth, except to protect caregivers during vaginal examinations or when the baby comes out of the vagina, due to the risk of HIV/AIDS.[2] It only serves to make childbirth seem more "medical." Putting masks on family members turns them into scared outsiders, afraid to intervene. This can be disheartening when you're trying to relax.

When are gowns and masks appropriate? In the operating room during a surgical procedure, such as a cesarean section, these garments are important to prevent infections caused by exposure to new germs and virulent germs carried in by strangers. There is one bacterium in particular that worries healthcare providers, beta-hemolytic streptococcus, but this will be screened for during good prenatal care. If a woman is known to have this microbe in her vagina, she will be given antibiotics when she comes to the hospital to prevent the baby from getting the same bacteria. But wearing gowns and masks does not prevent the presence of these bacteria.

You may not realize it, but your birth canal and your genitals are covered with healthy germs that do not need to be removed during birth, as your baby already has developed immunity to them from living inside your womb for the past nine months.

While hospitals typically provide birthing women with apparel on their arrival, feel free to ask if you can bring your own sleep attire— pajamas or a nightgown, a robe, and some slippers. You're going to be there for a while, and you should be comfortable.

When Is EFM Necessary?

Based on the scientific evidence, it's generally advisable to insist that there be no routine use (i.e., on all women) of electronic fetal monitoring during labor.[3] Why? The use of a monitor tends to initiate a cascade of additional interventions: A decision to speed up labor with drugs leads to the need for an epidural, which slows labor down and results in more frequent instrumental births, episiotomies, and cesareans. Furthermore, it can limit the freedom of movement that can be so critical to a woman's birth process. Of course, if a real complication develops, monitoring has proven value.

What exactly does an EFM do? In addition to measuring the strength and duration of uterine contractions, the device measures the speed of the baby's heartbeat, which, if it changes radically, could indicate distress. It cannot, however, measure the quality of the heartbeat, which is something for which a fetoscope is better suited. Imagine having a cardiologist who only read from an electrocardiogram and didn't bother to listen to the subtle murmurings of your heart before making a diagnosis. Wouldn't you probably switch physicians? Likewise, a machine cannot substitute for a skilled doctor's or midwife's hearing and discernment of what different sounds might indicate.

We know scientifically that the safest birth is a birth in which there is one-on-one continuous care from the same midwife or nurse throughout the labor and birth, a trained individual who monitors the birthing woman's condition and its various permutations through direct observation and frequent discussions about what the woman is feeling. Additionally, the same midwife or nurse will monitor the mother-to-be through frequent palpation of her abdomen and evaluation of her heart and the baby's heart, in addition to offering her emotional and physical care. The scientific evidence shows there is no improvement in outcomes with routine EFM of every woman in labor, although machines seem to be preferred to human monitoring in hospitals.[4] According to surveys, routine EFM for *all* birthing women is done in 8 percent of births in alternative birthing centers and 95 percent of hospital births. Research also shows that undergoing a screening EFM on admission doesn't improve the outcome.[5]

Why monitor labor? There is a real purpose in having someone watch what is going on, as things can start to go wrong in a few cases. If potential trouble is recognized early, it can be managed and prevented from becoming serious. There is clear evidence that having someone present who knows what to watch for all the time results in the best outcomes. This can be a midwife, a specially trained nurse, or a doctor.

In monitoring labor, attention must be paid not only to the fetal heart rate and the rate of the woman's uterine contractions (EFM does this), attention also needs to be paid to the condition of the woman in labor and the progress of labor (EFM doesn't do this). The progress of labor can be determined by carefully observing the condition of the woman and by doing occasional vaginal examinations to see how much the cervix is opening and how far down the birth canal the baby has come. If a trained person is present throughout labor, there truly is no need for EFM, as this trained person can listen to the fetal heart with a stethoscope, feel the uterine contractions with his or her hand, and at the same time note the condition of the woman and the progress of labor. This is the best and safest way to monitor normal birth. This is why routine monitoring with EFM is not recommended, even by ACOG, and in normal birth needs to be used only when trouble develops.

If a midwife or nurse or doctor is *not* going to be present with you at all times throughout labor, then intermittent use of an EFM can help the labor-and-delivery nurses in the hospital monitor what is going on. It is still essential that someone frequently come in to see how things are going with you and check the EFM strips. The EFM cannot replace frequent observation by a trained person using a stethoscope. Midwives today also use portable ultrasound machines called Dopplers as a means of monitoring.

Appropriate reasons for EFM include the following:

- *Induction or augmentation of labor:* If you are given a drug that jump-starts labor, speeds up labor, or "ripens" the cervix, you'll need constant electronic monitoring, as your contractions may be superstrong and affect the baby.

- *Too fast or too slow fetal heartbeat:* When signs of fetal distress are heard from listening with a stethoscope, using an electronic monitor is a good idea.

- *Baby in breech (feetfirst) position:* Potential complications deserve special ongoing attention.

When Are Intravenous (IV) Fluids Necessary?

In the old days, when childbirth was managed like gynecological surgery, a number of routines were carried out because they were routinely done when preparing a woman for an operation. These included giving her an enema, shaving her pubic hair, forbidding others from being in the room, putting a sterile gown and hat on the patient, requiring everyone in the room to wear a face mask, not allowing anything to be eaten or drunk for a number of hours before, putting the patient on her back on a table, and starting an IV.

As we have come to realize that childbirth is not gynecological surgery, these routines are gradually being dropped. Fortunately, there are no more enemas and pubic shaving of women in labor in U.S. hospitals. A limited number of visitors are now often allowed, although usually not children. More recently, routine IVs are in the process of being dropped—and this is good news as an IV can be unnecessary and ties a woman down.

If offered, you should refuse an IV unless you have a medical complication that requires it. The only times that an IV becomes necessary are as follows:

- *Dehydration:* This can occur from frequent vomiting and not drinking adequate fluids.

- *Inability to tolerate food:* As childbirth is strenuous and lasts for hours, women require nourishment to keep up their strength. On such occasions, they may need IV assistance. But this is not a routine requirement.

- *Epidural:* When you're being given this powerful pain medication, you'll need an IV simultaneously, because a fairly common risk with epidural is for a woman's blood pressure to suddenly drop precipitously due to the effect of the anesthetic drug on the spinal cord. Such a drop in maternal blood pressure means less blood gets to the baby, and so the baby often goes into distress from a lack of oxygen.

This cannot be allowed to continue as it could damage the baby. So the woman's blood pressure is closely watched and if it drops, a large quantity of IV fluid is given to the mother to counteract the falling blood pressure. This needs to be done quickly, and can be done more quickly if the IV catheter is already in place in the woman's arm.

When Is Lithotomy (the On-the-Back Position) Necessary?

A woman's freedom of movement should never be limited during childbirth. She needs to be able to shift position, walk, sit, or squat, and remain vertical as much as possible. The worst possible position in which a woman could labor is flat on her back. Except for when the woman is undergoing a surgical intervention, such as the rare justifiable extraction of the baby with vacuum or forceps, a doctor should never put a laboring woman on her back with her feet in stirrups.

Lithotomy is convenient for caregivers, but it is absolutely the worst position for facilitating the normal progress of labor and birth. Because the baby's head presses hard on the woman's aorta, the largest artery in her body, in this position—thus reducing blood flow to the baby—it is the position most likely to reduce the baby's oxygen supply. The so-called *semi-sitting position*, in which the woman is on her back with her upper body elevated by cranking the head of the bed up, is another wrong position for giving birth for the same reason.

There are certain complications for which it is an advantage to a doctor or midwife to put a woman in certain positions. For example, if there are signs of fetal hypoxia (oxygen deprivation) or distress, it can be useful to change the woman's position because the baby could possibly be compressing the umbilical cord. But if a woman or a baby is in trouble and needs special positions, it will almost always be a position on the mother's side—not her back. In fact, there is not a single complication in labor for which lithotomy is the best position. You should be off your back!

Normally a woman in labor needs to assume a vertical position: sitting, squatting, or standing. If your hospital doesn't have a birth stool, you may want to bring your own with you to the hospital—some models are small enough and light enough to be portable. Of course, consult with your hospital beforehand. This is also a good point to discuss with midwives and doulas.

Deborah Badran, a doula in New York City with fifteen years of experience, asserts: "In nearly all hospitals you lie down and they strap you into bed. So I ask if the laboring woman can sit up, and 'Can she stand up and cuddle?' If no one asks, it doesn't happen. But if someone suggests it and the staff can get the same readings, they let you. And it's a lot more comfortable way to handle pain, standing or sitting, than lying in a bed."

When Is Instrumental Birth Necessary?

Instrumentally assisted vaginal births are more common than they should be. They take place when the doctor thinks there is some urgent need to get the baby out fast, and either it needs to happen sooner than it would take to set up the operating room for a cesarean section, or the baby is so far descended in the birth canal that it appears easier to pull the baby out—extract it—than to push the baby back in and do a cesarean. As you'll recall from what happened in Natalie's story at the beginning of the chapter, sometimes extraction efforts don't succeed. In that case, her baby was too large to fit her birth canal.

Both forceps and vacuum extractors may be used to pull a baby quickly out of the mother's birth canal. Forceps are like oversized kitchen tongs. But instead of using this instrument to pick up an orange or serve salad, you put it around the head of the baby when it is still inside the woman—just before it comes out—and then you literally pull very hard to get the baby out. If it sounds primitive, that's because it is.

For a vacuum extractor, think of a big suction cup with a handle, like the plunger or plumber's helper that you use to unplug a toilet. You place the suction cup on the top of the head of the baby when it is still inside the mother—just before it comes out—and then the doctor literally pulls very hard to get the baby out. If it sounds primitive, well . . . it is.

Professionals choose either forceps or a vacuum extractor depending on the given situation. The vacuum has a lower (but not an absent) risk of damaging the baby's head and brain than the forceps and a lower (but not absent) risk of damaging the woman's vagina and genitalia.

An instrumental birth should be a rare situation—and it should only be a kind of desperate last-minute event because it can cause trauma to both the mother and the baby. But sadly there are still a few doctors out there who use forceps or vacuum extractors often for no good reason other than that they're in a hurry. The rare situations where extraction is necessary will never be more than about 0.5 percent to 2 percent.[6] This is not something you want to happen and you should not agree to it unless there is a true emergency. It is often a good idea to first try using the squatting position—called "midwives forceps." If instrumental extraction is proposed to you to be used by your doctor, your fully informed consent is essential.

Speed is a highly questionable reason to perform a vacuum extraction. Time doesn't matter as long as your baby is in good shape. Scientific research has shown that women receiving epidural block for normal labor pain have a significantly longer second stage of labor—just before the birth. This, in turn, results in a four times greater chance of a doctor recommending the use of forceps or vacuum extraction. But the evidence also shows that increased rates of pulling babies out with vacuum extractors or forceps is saving neither women's nor babies' lives. In 2002, babies were pulled out instrumentally in less than 1 percent of alternative birth-center births and 10 percent of hospital births.[7]

Legitimate reasons to consider instrumental birth include:

- *Fetal cord prolapse:* In this scenario, the umbilical cord gets caught around the baby as the baby descends through the birth canal. Eventually the cord is compressed and the umbilical blood supply is cut off so the baby receives no oxygen. The EFM will be showing severe, continuing fetal distress. Cesarean section is best unless the baby is too far down the birth canal.

- *Fetal distress that happens late in the birth:* Vacuum extraction is appropriate if fetal distress happens when the baby is already well descended into the birth canal, just before the head is about to come out. At this point, it is easier to quickly pull the baby out than to push the baby back in and do a cesarean section. A cesarean takes half an hour. Vacuum extraction takes only five or ten minutes. But if the baby is too far up the canal, this procedure is no use.

- *Oxygen deprivation:* Fetal extraction with vacuum or forceps may be necessary if there is clear evidence that the baby is oxygen deprived, such as might occur, for instance, when contractions are longer in duration than normal and there's too short a space of time between the contractions for an extended period.

If there is a real indication for instrumental vaginal birth, vacuum extraction is almost always preferred over forceps. Forceps are out of favor unless there's a rare technical reason to use them, such as that the baby already has a scalp electrode on. Evidence shows that there is a higher risk of damage to the birthing woman's vagina from forceps. Episiotomies, surgical incisions through the perineum (the tissue between the vagina and the rectum) to widen the vaginal opening (see chapter 8), are virtually guaranteed for assisted deliveries involving forceps or vacuum, both of which also cause short- and long-term harm to a woman's body. This type of intervention has serious proven risks for the mother, including possible urinary or fecal incontinence and painful intercourse. Plus, squeezing the baby's head can cause hemorrhages, skull fractures, and brain damage.

Valuable Questions

How can you avoid falling into the gap between what science has revealed are the best practices and what are the most commonly used, but flawed, medical practices? First, you need to get information ahead of time on the different interventions and technology that could be recom-

mended to you and weigh their potential benefits and risks. Read up on
them, using a critical eye. Second, request data on the past practices of
your doctor or midwife. For instance, what percentage of the birthing
women that your doctor (or midwife) has served ended up having instrumental births involving forceps or a vacuum extractor?

In considering whether or not a particular technology is appropriate
for your situation, it is also important that you understand the difference
between facts and value judgments. Every single technology has certain
benefits and certain risks. The chance that using it will make things better is its efficacy. The chance that using it will make things worse is its
risk. These are *facts* that can be scientifically measured. But benefit and
safety are value judgments about the *acceptability* of those chances. So, although your midwife or doctor can give you the facts on efficacy and
risk, as it is your body and your baby, only you can make the judgment
about acceptability. You must make a fully informed choice.

When a doctor or midwife suggests an intervention, either you or
an advocate (for example, a spouse, doula, friend, or close relative) may
ask the following questions on your behalf and help you interpret the
answers before you sign a consent form.

- Why do you want to use an EFM? (Or: IV, forceps, vacuum extractor, and so on)

- What are the medical indications for this intervention?

- Are there special considerations related to my special condition?

- What is the scientific evidence that this intervention (or technology)
  will make things better?

- What is the scientific evidence that this intervention (or technology)
  will make things worse?

- What are the risks to me of this intervention (or technology)?

- What are the risks to my baby of this intervention (or technology)?

- What are the long-term consequences?

• What are the short-term consequences?

• What are other possible solutions to the problem, including waiting longer?

• What are the risks and benefits of those alternate solutions?

• Why do you believe that using this intervention (or technology) has a better chance of success than not using it?

• What do you see happening to my baby and me if this intervention is not done?

• Is it possible to get a second opinion from another doctor or midwife on your suggestion?

The phrases "community standards" and "our standard of practice" only mean "This is how everyone does it here," which is an irrational and dangerous approach to medical practice. If you receive that kind of answer, be wary—you wouldn't drive ninety miles an hour on the freeway because others were. By rejecting any suggestion to put blind faith in what you are told you can or cannot do, you protect yourself and your baby. One way to get unbiased information is to insist on seeing the scientific data behind any information given to you. "Show me the data" is a powerful strategy for eliciting better information.

Adding Your Wishes to Your Birth Plan

Now that you've read this chapter, you are ready to consider what to put in your birth plan regarding technological interventions. It should be evident that we are talking in this section of the book about how you would prefer to manage unforeseeable events. Does technology have a role in your ideal normal, healthy, low-risk birth scenario? Maybe yes, maybe no. Under the care of a doctor in a hospital, high-tech interventions are plentiful, and you may not be able to avoid them entirely. Under the care of a midwife at home you may have limited access to technology. (In chapter 9, we'll survey the topic of high–risk birth.) If your labor had complications where would you stand on the issue of technology?

My hope is that you are able to use the information you've learned here as a basis for prelabor conversations with caregivers to elicit their practices and also to inform them, both orally and in writing, of how you wish to make decisions during labor. On a new page of your journal, reflect upon what you have learned about technology and how you feel about different interventions. Does this add new color to your previous plans?

In addition to technological devices you may encounter during birth (for better or worse), there is another kind of intervention that may be suggested by a doctor or a midwife—namely uterine-stimulating drugs and/or herbs. In the next chapter, we'll explore reasons why they're used, how effective they are, and possible consequences, and then you can add your wishes about these substances to your birth plan.

Ensuring the Appropriate Use of Drugs and Herbs

Induction and Augmentation

Former childbirth educator Leslie is the mother of six children whose births took various forms over three decades. Each and every time, she was under the care of a midwife. Yet the births took place in different settings: at home, in a birth center, and in a hospital. Her first child was born at home when she was in her twenties. Her last two children were born when she was in her forties. Although the second-to-last baby was born under low-key circumstances, Leslie herself decided she needed some support from medication. In her own words, "I had a lovely, appropriate use of Pitocin and epidural, which I would never have considered doing if I weren't that age. Administration was nicely done and we had a wonderful outcome. But anyone who tells you this is the same experience as natural birth is mistaken. You feel disconnected. It is medical—therefore you are treated differently."

Leslie decided to have the baby in a birth center located directly across the street from a hospital in her town in New England. She wanted to work with a midwife, and as she'd developed anemia during pregnancy, she also wanted to be near obstetric services in case of a complication like a hemorrhage. She knew that the midwives in the birth center had good relations with the hospital nurses. If anything happened, she wouldn't be caught in a professional crossfire.

Leslie's water broke at midnight and she checked herself in. She'd had one big contraction and then literally nothing was happening. She discussed it with her midwife, and they agreed that she would rest and make her decision later.

"When it got to be eight A.M.," says Leslie, "my feeling was, 'Let's get this show on the road!' Being an experienced mother, I knew how tired I felt and how inactive my uterus was behaving. My midwife was great. She asked, 'What do you want to do? We'll do whatever you want. You can try drinking herbal tea, nipple stimulation, or walking— you are welcome to do anything you want to start your labor.' Everyone left the choice up to me. When you make a choice, when you feel you have a choice, it makes a big difference. It makes you more confident. I checked with my intuition and said, 'I want Pitocin and an epidural.' I was sure I didn't want the first without the second."

Leslie had done postpartum counseling with many women who'd had a birth go wrong for one reason or another. Short of losing the baby, she saw that the loss of choice—either from what their bodies or the medical establishment did—was the factor that caused them the most emotional trouble and affected bonding with the baby. Thus Leslie knew that a woman has to do what she has to do. If Leslie ended up needing help, she wanted to view the experience as a success, rather than a failure. Empowerment was a goal. But, as she says, "The paradox is that at the moment when you're supposed to be empowered, you sometimes have to surrender your will for the betterment of the baby."

"I made the right choice for me. Because of the risk of staph infection after my water broke, and my anemia, the baby needed to come. I wasn't progressing. Remember, I'd been through this process four times already—I could tell the difference in the feeling of the early labor. Two hours later, at ten A.M., we called the anesthesiologist. I moved across the street to the hospital, where I was given the epidural and Pitocin, and an hour and a half later the baby was born. Every step I took was appropriate based on my informed consent and my understanding of my body and the procedures. The baby had no fetal distress, and I wasn't tired. He was protected and I was protected, because my labor was not long or drawn out. It is important to me that I made the choice."

Leslie points out, "After an epidural many women think, 'Why didn't I do natural childbirth?' The truth is, surviving pain and coping with it is golden. You could get that sense in another way, such as by writing a book or serving in the military. Natural birth may be the deepest route to the golden sense of self, since reproduction has been out of women's control for so long. I don't think there's anything more powerful you can do. Once you've done that, you realize you are in control of your own destiny. If you can make choices when you are most vulnerable, in pain, and another being is crashing out of your body, then you know that you can be strong and centered no matter what."

So when is it necessary in labor to use drugs or herbs, and how can you stay empowered when you choose to do so? This chapter will provide you with the information you need for deciding upon a safe birth for you and your child.

When Is Uterine Stimulation Necessary?

A woman's body is hormonally prepared over the nine-month gestation period to do what she would find impossible on an ordinary day. But in the climate that often surrounds childbirth, many women opt for taking drugs either to get labor started—worrying that they might have a "nonstarter" for a uterus—or to accelerate labor. Even when they feel that it's not ideal or suspect it could be inappropriate, many tolerate the medical approach to childbirth, as they believe they have no real choice—and because they are too often asked, "You don't want to take a chance with your baby, do you?" The lack of willingness on the part of some doctors, and even some midwives, to wait and let nature take its course is heartbreaking, as it prevents women from experiencing their bodies' astonishing power while exposing women and babies to all the dangers of these drugs.

According to the U.S. Centers for Disease Control and Prevention (CDC), the proportion of births in America that are induced, or "kick-started," by powerful drugs has more than doubled since 1989. Today, more than 40 percent of births are induced. It is also extremely common for labor to be augmented, or "speeded up," by drugs once it is already in progress. In addition, contractions are made so strong by these drugs that a woman's level of pain increases. From such statistics, you might conclude that women's bodies don't function properly. Of course, this simply isn't accurate. It's just that our culture doesn't seem to entirely trust women's bodies.

The truth is that complications during birth are less likely if your labor starts naturally, as your body "knows" when your baby is ready. Every day your baby remains in your uterus it grows bigger, stronger, and more developed.

Although the current induction rate in the United States is more than 40 percent, adding up the valid reasons to induce labor accounts for only about 5 percent of pregnancies.[1] Let's look at what constitutes an appropriate reason.

- *The baby is significantly overdue:* The big issue today in induction of labor is at what point to induce labor when the pregnancy has gone beyond the normal due date of forty weeks' gestation. After that a pregnancy is considered "postterm." Of course, it's important to remember that birth doesn't actually happen on a specific day, but rather *around* that day. Spontaneous birth any time in the period between thirty-seven weeks and forty-two weeks is a perfectly normal variation. After forty-two weeks a baby may be considered overdue, and it would be reasonable to watch closely and wait as well as consider inducing labor. Before forty-two weeks you should only induce if there are definite signs that the baby is in trouble.[2]

- *Placental malfunction:* Like everything else, the placenta has a life cycle. It grows and then ultimately gets older and older with decreasing functions. There is normal variation in this cycle. Some placentas are old at forty weeks. Others aren't yet old at forty-four weeks. On a bell-shaped curve, more than 95 percent of all placentas can still function normally at forty-two weeks. As the placenta ages, it begins to function more poorly, so less oxygen and nutrition are reaching the baby. Evidence of placental malfunction, such as that the baby stops growing or the baby isn't moving around as much as it should be, is a good reason for induction.

• *The baby is too small for its gestational age:* This can be a sign of placental malfunction, and a situation in which induction may be warranted.

• *Preeclampsia:* Usually occurring in mid to late pregnancy, preeclampsia is a condition characterized by high blood pressure and excessive protein in the urine, swelling, weight gain, nausea, headaches, and vision changes. It indicates tremendous strain on the mother's body and toxicity, and therefore induction may be appropriate. A mild elevation in blood pressure without any of these other symptoms is common late in pregnancy and is not justification for induction. It's a good idea to get a second opinion.

• *Water breaks:* The amniotic sac, or "membranes," provides a barrier to germs that keeps the baby sterile during pregnancy. If the amniotic sac is broken either spontaneously, as frequently occurs just before labor or early in labor, or by being ruptured artificially by the doctor or midwife, as is sometimes done to stimulate labor, then the protective barrier is gone. Bacteria can slowly ascend up the vagina into the uterus and potentially cause infection. Once the amniotic sac has ruptured, there is an increased threat of infection, your caregiver should keep vaginal exams to a minimum. However, watchful waiting is a good approach that is underused. With no signs of infection, it is usually safe to wait at least forty-eight hours before considering induction.

• *The baby is showing signs of oxygen deprivation (fetal hypoxia):* If the baby starts showing signs of distress, taking measures to accelerate labor may be a good idea. An electronic fetal monitor should be hooked up and its strips followed closely. Getting a second opinion on the reading of the paper strip that comes from the fetal monitor is always a good idea. Reading the information recorded by the monitor takes training, experience, and a great deal of interpretation. The ability to interpret these electronic scribbles varies widely among obstetricians and labor-and-delivery nurses. In practice, there is a high rate of false positive readings for fetal distress. In other words, the tracing on the paper is interpreted as showing fetal distress when there is none.

For situations such as these, obstetricians can and do prescribe drugs, such as Pitocin, which has a long history of use and is FDA approved. When labor must be augmented, midwives—like doctors—may rely upon Pitocin to stimulate uterine contractions. However, midwives tend to be more conservative about how soon they'll step in.

Questionable reasons to consider inducing or augmenting labor, often unjustified, include:

• *The baby is too big (macrosomia):* Unless there are signs of a malfunctioning placenta, the size of the baby is not an adequate reason to jump-start labor. If the mother is in some way disfigured or structurally unable to deliver the baby vaginally, allowing the baby its full period of gestation nonetheless fosters the baby's good health, after which a cesarean may become necessary (see chapter 8).

Think about it logically. Babies' heads are soft and malleable, and do not fully harden until many weeks after birth for a reason: so the baby's head can be gradually molded to fit safely through the birth canal. The mother's cervix, when softened (ripened) and fully dilated, is enormously stretchy, too. Macrosomia has been used as an excuse for induction, but the data do not support it.[3] Indeed, trying to induce labor with a large baby by stimulating contractions with induction drugs is contraindicated with macrosomia, as it might harm both the mother and the baby.

• *Gestational diabetes:* Recent research has shown that there is no such thing as gestational diabetes.[4] It is perfectly normal for a woman to undergo changes in the metabolism of sugar during her pregnancy. After all, her hormones are shifting and her body is nourishing the body of a second, developing person.

• *Too much (or too little) amniotic fluid in the bag of waters:* In actuality, the bag of waters prevents the baby from pressing and slamming against the mother's bones during pregnancy, and especially during labor. It protects both the mother and her baby from harm. Thus, it's better not to rupture it. In very rare situations, abnormal levels of amniotic fluid volume can cause pressures and problems. But the present ultrasound scanning tests to measure amniotic fluid volume are quite crude, and the results of the tests are questionable unless they are extremely low or high, which is a rare outcome. This would be an extremely unlikely complication, and one that would almost never justify induction. If induction is recommended on the basis of too much or too little amniotic fluid, you can ask for tests that measure fetal well-being and request a second opinion.

• *Failure to progress:* "Failure to progress" is a label adhered to the birth experience that has the potential to initiate a slippery slope of interventions, including the most extreme of all, cesarean section. It basically means, "This process is taking too long." This is a common excuse given to augment the labor with drugs and is the most common excuse of all given for cesarean section. "Failure to progress" is a concept reflecting the idea that there is a need to be in a hurry during labor and birth when the latest and best obstetric textbooks, after a thorough review of the evidence, state emphatically that, in fact, there is no prescribed length of time for the different stages of labor (see chapter 1).[5] Yet, many hospitals still hang clocks on the wall and watch them closely. If a woman is in second-stage labor for more than two hours, an alarm is raised and interventions commence. However, such measures aren't usually warranted. Suffice it to say that in a major study of 5,000 births in the United States, eighty-two mothers were in second-stage labor for more than six hours and none had trouble.[6] Their babies were A-OK.

Understanding Drugs and Herbs

The human body is a chemical factory. Chemical reactions keep us warm, make it possible for us to move, and so forth. Food is actually composed of chemicals (such as vitamins, minerals, amino acids, sugars, and, yes, fats) that we require to function. Digestion separates these chemicals and the blood circulates them through the body. We eliminate the ones we don't need, and those we have used up, by breathing and sweating them out and excreting them in our urine and feces.

Drugs and herbal remedies are chemicals that have been shown to alter the chemistry in the body in a beneficial way. This takes many forms. For instance, if a chemical is missing from the body, such as insulin in the case of diabetes, the drug insulin replaces that missing chemical. If a chemical reaction in the body has gone haywire, such as they do in cancer, a drug may block that chemical reaction.

For a drug or herb to be beneficial, it must be given in just the right amount or it may alter the body chemistry in a different way than anticipated. Then it would no longer be beneficial, and might even be harmful—poisonous. (Poisons are substances that block chemical reactions essential to our lives.) Every drug or herb has the potential to make the chemistry of the body better or to make it worse.

Which Drugs Are Commonly Encountered in Labor and Birth?

The drugs commonly given to women during childbirth include antibiotics, uterine stimulants, and pain medications. Pain medication—analgesics and nerve blocks—will be covered in chapter 7. Let's discuss the two other types of medications here.

- *Antibiotics:* Antibiotics should not be given during labor and birth unless there is a definite indication for them as they may pass through the placenta to the baby—see below.

One indication is the presence of a bad bacterium called beta-hemolytic streptococcus. These germs can sometimes reside in the woman's vagina during pregnancy without making the woman sick, but are dangerous if the baby comes in contact with them. A screening test can detect these dangerous bacteria, and if present, the woman should be treated with antibiotics before and/or during birth in order to prevent them from infecting the baby as it passes through the birth canal. Once the water breaks, and if it has been more than forty-eight hours since the rupture of the membranes, antibiotics are usually started as a precautionary measure.

Another indication for antibiotics during labor is when a woman develops signs of infection, usually a fever. As a low-grade fever can be a normal result of all the hard work the woman is doing during labor, a blood test may be done for confirmation. If it reveals further signs of infection, antibiotics are started. The fever may be due to infection in the placenta or uterus, and this condition requires treatment.

• *Uterine stimulants:* These drugs are used to induce labor that has not started and—for an important medical reason—needs to start, or to augment contractions if labor has started but is seriously slowing down or has stopped.

There are three types of drugs known to stimulate uterine contractions. The first and safest is oxytocin, a hormone normally released in the body in certain situations, such as during sexual arousal and breastfeeding, which is artificially synthesized and manufactured under the brand name Pitocin for intramuscular or intravenous use. The second type is prostaglandin 2, another hormone normally released in the body in certain situations, which is artificially synthesized and manufactured by two different pharmaceutical companies for use as a vaginal suppository. One company sells it by the brand name Cervidil. The other company markets it as Prepidil.

The third type of uterine stimulant that has come into common use in the past decade is another artificially synthesized prostaglandin called misoprostol, or prostaglandin 1. This drug is manufactured as a pill and sold under the name Cytotec for oral use in treating stomach ulcers. As an unintentional side effect it produces uterine contractions. The Food and Drug Administration (FDA) has not approved it for use in pregnant women.

Warning: Pregnant women should never consent to the use of Cytotec to induce or augment labor. If this drug is suggested to you before or during labor, ask your physician to show you the package insert containing the manufacturer's warnings and you'll immediately read that this practice is nonapproved for "off-label" use, which has previously been the cause of extreme and catastrophic uterine ruptures. The warning even has a visual image of a pregnant woman in silhouette inside a circle with a diagonal line through it.

The FDA has approved Pitocin, Cervidil, and Prepidil for stimulating uterine contractions, based on reliable research studies.[7] Cytotec has never been approved for stimulating uterine contractions, and it has never been adequately studied for this purpose. Most of the "research" results are either anecdotal or studies with far too few women involved to make valid measure of risks possible. These results are then passed around between doctors informally.

How Are Drugs Evaluated?

Since drugs can be either beneficial or harmful, it is essential to evaluate them before they are used. Usually studies are done first on animals and then on humans who have volunteered for research. This evaluation includes the determination of the best dose and best way of administration, and also important ways to reduce the risks and keep risks to a minimum. If the evaluation determines that, in most cases, the benefits outweigh the risks, the drug may be approved for use with labeling to inform both the healthcare provider and the patient of potential benefits, risks, and means of administration.

When someone offers you a drug during childbirth, you need to be on the alert. If you're like most parents, the birth of your baby is the last situation in which you'd knowingly choose to participate in a pharmacological experiment! Use the valuable questions on pages 101–102 as your guide in speaking with medical personnel.

How Safe Is Uterine Stimulation with Drugs?

Drug-induced labor comes with real risks for a woman and her baby. Scientific evidence shows that drugs may or may *not* accelerate labor, while they definitely increase the number of additional interventions that women undergo.[8] Nonetheless, this procedure is being sold to women as safe, and in the process is proving to be an enormous convenience to doctors and hospitals. Is the convenience worth it? Are the risks low or high? Let's see.

- *Maternal death:* There is a very low risk of maternal mortality in wealthy countries. But it has been increasing in the United States now for more than fifteen years, and the increasing number of American women dying during pregnancy and childbirth is almost certainly related to the increasing rates of induction of labor and cesarean section (see chapter 6). Why should induction of labor lead to the woman dying? Because evidence shows that the use of the uterine stimulants for induction of labor sharply increases the risk of a rupture of the uterus. This carries a significant risk of maternal death and also leads to amniotic fluid embolism—a condition from which 80 percent of the women die.[9] Risk has two elements. First, how frequently does what's being risked happen? Second, how bad is it when it happens? Uterine rupture and amniotic fluid embolism are rare, but when they happen they are a disaster with high rates of maternal mortality.

- *Fetal brain damage and mortality:* There is good scientific evidence that induction with drugs frequently causes the uterus to contract too fast,[10] and considerable evidence that such hyperstimulation during labor can lead to a baby with severe, permanent brain damage—and in some cases fetal death.[11] Why? The only time the baby can get oxygen from the mother during labor is the period between uterine contractions. If the uterus contracts too often, there is no chance for the baby to get enough oxygen. In addition, induction of labor with uterine stimulant drugs increases the risk, as discussed just above, of both uterine rupture and amniotic fluid embolism, and both of these complications carry a high risk of fetal and newborn death.

- *Increased likelihood of instrumental and surgical birth:* Another undesirable spin-off of induction is that it leads to more babies being pulled out of their mothers with forceps or a vacuum extractor (see chapter 5) and more babies being cut out of their mothers with cesarean section (see chapter 8). All such births carry increased risks for both women and babies.

- *Interferes with bonding and breastfeeding:* It alters the mother's hormones.

Which Herbs Are Commonly Encountered in Labor and Birth?

For thousands of years before pharmaceutical medications became available, herbs were gathered and cultivated around the world for medicinal purposes. Among other uses, plant medicine has a long history of benefiting childbearing women, and today some midwives continue this tradition. If you work with a midwife, herbs may be suggested to you for two main purposes: to soften and prepare the cervix to open and to boost labor.

Evening primrose oil is one of a few natural remedies that you might encounter under the care of a midwife that may help soften your cervix. Sometimes it is given orally, and other times it is applied directly to the cervix. As with drugs, it doesn't always have the effect someone hopes it will. Black cohosh is another herb often used to prepare a woman's cervix for childbirth. *Be advised: You must be cautious when using an herb for this purpose not to use it too early in pregnancy, as you want pregnancy to last full term. Consult your midwife for professional help in making a determination.*

Native Americans have used blue cohosh for centuries to strengthen the action of the uterus, jump-start a stalled uterus, and ease labor pains. Many midwives recommend a special combination of herbs called PN6 to their clients in the final weeks of pregnancy, which includes the ingredients of red raspberry leaves, squaw vine, blessed thistle, black co-hosh, and false unicorn root, as well as omega-3 fats.

If you are considering herbs recommended by a midwife, just the same as you would with a drug, you need to weigh the potential benefits of the herbs against their potential adverse side effects, such as gastrointestinal distress, headaches, dizziness, and so on; and you need to investigate the contraindications, such as high blood pressure, drug interactions, and so forth. Make certain that anyone who advocates taking herbs is well educated in both the herbs' actions and their contraindications. To evaluate a practitioner's herbal knowledge, ask where the person learned about herbs—does this individual have professional accreditation?—and what the person's past experience in applying their knowledge of herbs has been. Ask to see research on recommended herbs, and feel free to seek a second opinion.

How Are Herbs Evaluated?

Herbs are marketed in the United States as food supplements and are not required to go through as rigorous a screening process as drugs, as long as their manufacturers do not make specific, unsupported health claims for their usage. They are not completely unregulated, however. Producers are required to produce uniform doses, for instance, so consumers know what they are getting.

Although the difference between drugs and herbs is somewhat arbitrary, a general difference is that drugs are artificially produced while herbs are naturally occurring. Having said this, some of our most important drugs—penicillin, digitalis (the important heart drug), and many others—occur in nature and the WHO operates a program that combs the earth looking for naturally occurring drugs. As most drugs are artificially synthesized or, if they occur naturally, are prepared in a laboratory for use as drugs, they are included in the system of scientific evaluation.

By and large, anyone can get their hands on herbs and it is only quite recently that attempts are being made to scientifically evaluate them. Companies tend not to invest in research on herbs, because these are nonproprietary substances, meaning they cannot be patented, or exclusively owned, so research would help both them and their competitors.

Do Drugs and Herbs Given to the Mother Cross the Placenta?

The dependence of the fetus on the mother for essential nutrients places the fetus at the mercy of the placenta when foreign substances such as drugs and herbs appear in the mother's blood. For example, the consequences of maternal alcohol ingestion, cigarette smoking, and cocaine use on fetal growth and development are now well documented. To consider the placenta a barrier to drugs is not correct. The fetus is to some extent exposed to essentially all substances taken by the mother. The question is not *if* drugs cross the placenta, but *the rate* at which they do so.

Most antibiotics are known to cross the placental barrier, although the rate at which they do so varies. However, enzymes in the placenta usually change drugs that are naturally occurring hormones (for example, oxytocin and the prostaglandins), or are closely related synthetic variants, so that these drugs are not a threat to the fetus.

Because the placenta is a highly permeable organ, limiting the use of drugs and herbs during pregnancy and childbirth has long been recommended. This is why drugs used on women during pregnancy and birth need special evaluation. A pharmaceutical company wishing to get FDA approval for use of a drug during pregnancy and/or birth is mandated to do studies on pregnant and birthing women. Therefore, it is perfectly appropriate to ask to see the research and to expect the results to be readily available.

Valuable Questions

It is best to investigate the drugs and/or herbs that may be suggested to you before you go to the hospital to give birth, as some are controversial. In creating your birth plan, it is a good idea to find out which drugs and herbs your primary care provider uses most commonly, and then make a judgment about them based on the balance between benefit and risk.

If during labor or birth your doctor or midwife suggests a drug or herb, insist they give you the full information. Ask to read the drug's package insert. And, if it is feasible, go online (or ask a family member or friend to go online for you) and gather information. Remember, except in cases of emergency, you have plenty of time to make a decision. There is a lot of hanging around and waiting in the early stages of labor.

Caution: Not all Internet sites are equal. When looking for valid research results, seek them from major institutions, as these are most reliable. Try the National Institutes of Health or Centers for Disease Control and Prevention websites, for instance (see Resources).

Here is a list of questions you may ask your primary care provider when either induction or augmentation with drugs or herbs is being suggested to you.

- Why are you suggesting induction (or augmentation)?

- What are the medical indications for it?

- Is this use of this drug approved by the FDA?

- Are there special considerations related to my specific condition?

- What is the scientific evidence that this drug (or herb) will make things better?

- What is the scientific evidence that this drug (or herb) will make things worse?

- What are the risks to me?

- What are the risks to my baby?

- What are the short-term consequences?

- What are the long-term consequences?

- How often do your patients need an epidural after taking this drug (or herb)?

- How often do your patients need instrumental births after taking this drug (or herb)?

- How often do your patients need a cesarean section after taking this drug (or herb)?

- What are other possible solutions?

- What are the risks and benefits of those alternate solutions?

- What do you see happening if I do not take this drug (or herb)?

Creative Alternatives to Encourage Labor

If the uterus must be encouraged to contract at the beginning or in the middle of labor, it is important to remember that this effect often can be achieved without turning to powerful and sometimes risky drugs. First, there is the completely natural method of sexual stimulation, which triggers the release of the hormone oxytocin and causes the uterus to contract. The effect can be achieved through nipple stimulation, clitoral stimulation, or by another means of sexual arousal.

Interestingly, semen contains natural prostaglandins, and so having unprotected sex with your sexual partner, if he ejaculates inside you, might also trigger labor to commence. If your water has broken, this is not a good strategy, of course. However, for a postterm baby being carried by a healthy mother, it couldn't hurt. (At the very least, it can distract you.)

Long walks and other forms of gentle exercise are another means of speeding labor along. Gravity is your friend, as it brings the pressure of the baby to bear on the parts of your body that need to relax and open up. Eating spicy food is yet another folk remedy for inducing labor. So here you have the makings of a great date: a Mexican dinner, followed by a long walk, and lovemaking—followed by having a baby!

Adding Your Wishes to Your Birth Plan

When it comes to medication, a lay consumer, such as you, of course has to rely on the advice of those who have more experience and knowledge. But your caregivers owe you a good explanation and part of their job is to help you make sense of potential problems. That's informed consent. Let me reiterate that most complications in labor come on gradually so there is enough time to weigh your decisions and respond appropriately. At this step in creating your birth plan, you are planning for contingencies, as you were when you worked through the topic of technology in the last chapter. Under what conditions would you feel comfortable with inducing/augmenting labor? Write about it in your journal.

Also consider this: How conservative is your caregiver about offering pregnant women and women in labor drugs or herbs? What statistics of usage have you been given by your doctor or midwife? What are the policies of the hospital or out-of-hospital birth center about the duration of labor? You may wish to go back and reevaluate earlier sections of your birth plan based on the new information you've learned.

Another matter that must be carefully weighed before you go into labor is the use of strong medication—epidurals and analgesics—to manage labor pain. Many pregnant women, especially first-time moms, are afraid of confronting natural labor pain. And many women haven't learned what you know now: that artificial acceleration of labor makes contractions stronger and harder to tolerate without relief. In the next chapter, we'll talk about pain-management strategies, including several nondrug options.

Seven

What You Need to Know About Pain Management

Relaxation Techniques, Ambiance, and Epidurals

At thirty-two, Dana was eager to give birth to her child. A former dancer, she was highly attuned to her physical condition and recognized her body's capacity to perform under pressure. "In our culture, we work hard at the gym for less important reasons. When pain came from the different pressures inside my body, I was waiting to open to creation, to unfold. I wanted my baby so much. How could I not embrace this dimension of my body?" Dana was hoping for a natural birth and chose to be in a hospital so she could feel free to dance, scream, and perhaps curse without offending the neighbors. Part of Dana's planning process was to practice meditation.

When Dana's water broke, she and her husband went to the hospital. Since there wasn't a place in maternity for Dana yet, for the next twenty-four hours she and her husband sat in a group ward with women bedridden by complications from pregnancy. It wasn't nice being there, but they were well prepared so that nothing would stop the flow of intimacy between them. They decided they would create a happy reality for themselves.

If a woman's water breaks, the policy of the hospital was to put her on antibiotics after twelve hours and to induce labor after twenty-four hours if there was no dilation. Although Dana wanted a natural birth, she quickly made a decision not to fight the doctors. "If I chose to fight, I would suffer," she says, "whereas if I went with the drugs, I would enjoy the birth no matter what happened."

Dana's solution was to give in with happiness, receiving the antibiotics with open arms. She was having mild contractions, but was not dilating much. At 3 A.M. on Thursday, she was moved to the delivery room and given Pitocin. She says, "Once you receive this, the contractions are at the hardest level. A natural delivery slowly builds in intensity, but when you get this drug you go immediately to the most painful place."

Despite the intensity, Dana reports, "It was still the most beautiful thing I've ever experienced. And the most beautiful experience I could ever imagine with my partner." Dana did her best to be comfortable. She bounced and circled on a Pilates ball just to keep moving. When the contractions came she leaned on the bed or her husband.

After jumping and moving for nine hours, the opening of her cervix was only four centimeters large. The hospital midwife who came on duty around that time approached Dana about having an epidural. (Usually women can't naturally handle the pain of the contractions that come with the Pitocin.) Thirty-three hours into being there and not having slept the night before her water broke, Dana was still reluctant.

"I thought, 'I can get the epidural now or I can ask for the Pitocin and the monitor to be turned off. I can sign a form saying I am responsible for my birth and go on with a natural birth, but that means fighting the situation,' which is what I decided not to do. . . . In that deep space, I nourished and loved the doubt that came in. Having the doubt allowed me to see the whole picture clearly: I could fight or work with the givens. I blessed the givens. From the deepest state of meditation I felt the fatigue and how truly exhausted I was, and I heard a deep voice saying, 'Take the epidural.' So I knew the medication was right for me.

"I took the epidural and it was the only time I didn't feel anything. That was the only moment that fear truly came into my heart! It was scary not to feel labor, even more frightening than feeling pain. But again I did a relaxation and said, 'OK, just enjoy.' Fifteen minutes later I went to sleep with my husband lying near me on the bed.

"Two hours later, the contractions woke me up. I was fully awake, filled with new, full strength. It had been truly refreshing. I called the anesthesiologist and asked him to release the epidural. He closed the nozzle so I could stand again and dance. Now the monitor and epidural were both out of me. It was the most beautiful thing to feel pain again after being numb."

After a half an hour, Dana's cervix dilated to five centimeters. Fifteen minutes later, she felt the baby's head dropping down. She was at six centimeters. Within a few minutes she went from being halfway there to all the way there. At nine centimeters, the midwife said, "OK, we're in delivery." The room changed. The staff took out sterilized objects and made room for the midwife to work. Dana was laughing and talking to her baby for the next twenty minutes. Nothing mattered to her but to focus on the baby and to be with her on her way out. When the baby's head was out, she opened her eyes and was watching.

"I can truly say from the deepest place in my heart, there wasn't an inch of time, not a piece of time that I would give up from the whole process. With every contraction I got closer and closer to my husband in a way I didn't know I could be and more prepared for whatever would come. A mother is coming to the world, a father is coming to the world, and a family is coming to the world. This was how we were born."

The Pain-Pleasure Paradigm

Women feel varying degrees of pain and euphoria during normal, healthy childbirth. In fact, as the authors of *A Guide to Effective Care in Pregnancy and Childbirth* so aptly state, "Satisfaction in childbirth is not contingent upon the absence of pain."[1] Although it is rarely discussed in the mainstream literature, some women—perhaps as many as 20 percent by informal estimates—experience painless, even orgasmic pleasure during drug-free labor. Frequently the euphoria coexists with pain, as in Dana's case, for as the intensity of labor builds a woman's body releases adrenaline, which boosts her endurance, and endorphins, natural stress-reducing hormones that take the edge off pain.

Your beliefs and expectations about pain and childbirth, the personal goals you've set for motherhood, your earlier life experiences, and your previous experiences in giving birth may factor significantly into the upcoming experience. However, in creating your birth plan, as of today—or at least soon—you can begin taking charge of your attitudes, emotions, and responses to any pain you may undergo. To prepare yourself physically, mentally, and emotionally ahead of time, you can take steps such as attending a class on childbirth, doing prenatal yoga or stretching, and learning to meditate or do self-hypnosis.

Some women perceive childbirth as an empowering challenge or a lesson, and this enables them to tolerate normal discomfort. Other women fear giving birth for one major reason: They don't know if they can endure its strong sensations. They worry about permanent harm or being traumatized. Of course, their stress and anxiety only promote tension, a state counterproductive to giving birth. Making proactive choices helps.

Aspects of the environment you are in can modify and ease your pain, too, and so can the support you receive from your caregivers and companions. There are many ways to create favorable conditions. Particularly in the early stages of labor, even before a pain-relieving drug may be safely administered, all women can benefit from preparation.

Certainly, unless your caregivers identify medical contraindications, you also have the option of receiving an epidural to block your pain toward the end of labor. What factors other than pain should be weighed when anesthesia is being offered? In this chapter, we'll consider the pros and cons of this popular pain medication, along with self-empowerment techniques such as self-hypnosis, visualization, breathing, meditation, relaxation, and prayer. We'll discuss numerous ways of reducing and eliminating tension during healthy birth, so you feel more confident going through this powerful experience.

Before we do, let's consider the physiological purpose that pain serves.

Childbirth Pain as a Feedback Mechanism

Why is there pain in normal labor? Even though we don't love it, pain is not a negative. Rather it is a messenger. Stick your finger into fire and the pain you feel will immediately make you withdraw it for your own protection. As you saw in chapter 2, childbirth is orchestrated by a woman's brain through her autonomic nervous system, the part that is not under her conscious control. This system regulates physical processes such as heart rate, body temperature, and digestion. Although you may be aware of your stomach and intestines working, you don't oversee the digestive work, right? So it is with childbirth.

A woman's contracting uterus and her stretching cervix and vagina send pain impulses to her brain that she may interpret as a useless byproduct, instead of an integral part of her experience. In reality, these impulses result in the release of key hormones into the bloodstream that carry messages back to a woman's body and ensure that labor progresses normally. These impulses also guide a woman to shift position and do whatever else she must to facilitate the birth process. If we interrupt this feedback loop by blocking her pain impulses, a woman's labor can slow, or even stop, at which point it becomes necessary to intervene using uterine stimulants, forceps or vacuum extraction, and/or cesarean section. All interventions carry some risks for mother and baby.

That being said, pain is not pleasant and it can be frightening, therefore it must be managed intelligently. The less tense you are and the less scared, the less pain there will be to overcome and the easier it will be to cope with birth. Getting educated about childbirth, being familiar with your body and its sensations, and communicating these to your birth attendants is important, as they can check you and determine whether or not everything is progressing normally. If it is, they can offer you reassurance and comfort. If not, they can intervene in a timely manner with instruments or surgery. Pain informs everyone involved about the appropriate management of labor.

Excruciating pain, such as sharp or burning pain, is a very different kind of pain than the sensation of having a strong labor contraction. If you communicate terrible or abnormal sensations to your birth attendants, the nurses and your midwife or doctor know how to check that your baby is descending appropriately through the birth canal. Unfortunately, after having an epidural a woman would not feel even the most searing pain indicating that something had gone critically wrong. I have seen a few cases in which there was a serious delay in diagnosing a uterine rupture because the woman had received an epidural. The important function pain plays as messenger was lost.

By planning ahead, you can clearly communicate how you feel to your attendants during your labor, even if it means that ultimately you may have to decide to abandon your plans in favor of a new course of action. You could be surprised to discover that a sensation that alarms you at first is actually quite normal.

Pain Is a Matter of Perception

In *Ina May's Guide to Childbirth*, acclaimed midwife Ina May Gaskin cites a 1988 cross-cultural study of Dutch and American women who gave birth in hospitals, asking about their expectations of pain and whether or not they used medication. "Both the Dutch group and the U.S. group were informed of the potential negative effects of pain-relieving medications for labor. Nearly two-thirds of the Dutch group received no pain medication, in contrast with only one-sixth of the U.S. women. Two-thirds of the U.S. group were given narcotics during labor, along with some type of nerve block for birth."[2]

Here's the kicker: "The U.S. women *expected* labor to be more painful than the Dutch women did, and they expected to be given medication for pain. In both groups, the proportions of women expecting pain to those who received medication were nearly identical." In other words, this relatively small sampling demonstrates that internal attitudes factor heavily into the birth experience and are partly responsible for the degree of medication that women require—and any consequences of taking that medication.

Apparently people have different pain thresholds, levels at which they are personally unwilling to surpass and endure. No, there are no merit badges handed out for enduring pain; however, given the risks associated with pain medication and given that the pain can inform a woman and caregiver of how well or poorly the birth is progressing, if you can handle the pain of childbirth through another means than drugs, it would be advisable. Pain is a normal feedback mechanism in the body that regulates the progress of labor.

Less invasive and far safer methods of effective pain management than an epidural include—in no particular order—freedom of movement, continuous presence of the same companion or birth attendant, water immersion, self-hypnosis, counterpressure, and massage. Also bear in mind that labor pain is significantly increased by laboring in an unfamiliar place, being surrounded by unfamiliar people (or being left alone), lying in a horizontal position, not being allowed to move, having membranes artificially ruptured, and having induction or augmentation with drugs. Many women request epidurals after other procedures are done that increase their pain, which is why epidural rates in American hospitals are high.

While you are likely to find that hospital personnel define pain as an evil to be stamped out with potent drugs, midwives in planned out-of-hospital births—taking place in alternative birth centers or at home—understand that labor pain has a physiological function and can be relieved with scientifically proven, nonpharmacological methods, beginning with general measures for coping with the triggers for natural anxiety.

Coping with Your Anxiety
⟶◌

Heidi Rinehart, M.D., an obstetrician formerly affiliated with the Northern New Mexico Women's Health and Birth Center, says, "First-time moms are generally anxious about two things. First, how can the baby come out without them being torn from stem to stern? Second, they're anxious because it's a new experience, like going to high school, taking a test, or getting a job. They hope they're going to do OK. That's only natural.

"Women have other fears; for instance, if they've been sexually abused, because they've had trauma to the vagina, or have endured battering. Or they're afraid because they've known someone who died in childbirth. All these women need extra gentleness and understanding to help them figure out, 'How can I approach this confidently?'"

Herself a mother, Rinehart asserts, "The human body is incredible, which is one of the things that's so cool about having a baby naturally. There are the same kind of rewards and sense of accomplishment in childbirth as for those who run marathons. After a baby, a woman can say, 'I've pushed myself farther than I've gone before. I'm stronger than I gave myself credit. No matter what I do that's hard and challenging, I can look back at childbirth and know if I could do that, then surely I can do this.' Birth is an affirming, challenging experience that shows women how strong they are. It's the same reason people climb to the top of Mt. Everest. Because I've had two babies, I don't need to climb a mountain to know how patient, persevering, and strong I am. I already know it."

An overriding factor in a woman's ability to relax and calmly respond to all kinds of different events that confront her in labor is if she has the confidence to navigate the experience. Whether it's her first or fifth child, a woman who knows how to approach birth as transformative and empowering is more relaxed. The more informed women are, the more relaxed they feel. Relaxation partly has to do with the kind of person you are.

In the classic 1959 book *Childbirth Without Fear*, British obstetrician

Grantly Dick-Read described how anxiety makes pain worse. When a woman in labor is fearful, her mind informs her body that there's danger. As the body protectively interprets this as a need to prevent the baby from being born, her body tenses. The inside layer of her uterus becomes rigid, even as other muscles aim to expel the baby. Her body is resisting itself. Pain develops, the woman gets tenser, and the birth can be very painful.

Do older or younger women feel more anxiety? Older women can be less anxious than young women because they already know themselves and what to do to call upon their resources. But if any woman, old or young, has had a very rough first birth experience, she may have a much higher level of anxiety going into another birth. Younger mothers have anxiety because they've never been through birth. But they tend not to have been traumatized by a birth either, so sometimes they are more relaxed about their births.

Techniques for Natural Pain Relief

Even if you ultimately have an epidural as Dana did, you cannot escape pain entirely. It is important not to have an epidural too early in labor (before your cervix has reached a dilation of four or five centimeters) or it will literally stop the labor. Therefore, there will be several hours of pain before you can consider seeking relief from an epidural. You may be given other pain medication, but nothing that blocks the nerves. Please understand: Every pharmacological method poses real risks for you and your baby. It's important to learn what the risks are so that you can make the most informed choices for your situation.

By far the most effective means to control pain in labor is through the love and personal attention of others. That's a scientifically proven fact. Here are several other nondrug techniques for natural pain management.

- *Movement:* Left to their own devices, most laboring women spontaneously shift their bodies to adapt to changing conditions, moving until they achieve some relief from their discomfort. As Murray Enkin and his coauthors of *A Guide to Effective Care in Pregnancy and Childbirth* write: "When the mother changes position, she alters the relationship between gravity, uterine contractions, the fetus, and her pelvis."[3] Much of what a woman feels depends on the size of her baby and where it is pressing, her womb shape and skeletal structure, and the strength of her contractions. Walking, dancing, bouncing on a birth ball, hanging from a support bar, leaning forward, squatting, and getting onto your hands and knees are only a few positions that you may find relieve the pain of labor (see chapter 2 for more suggestions).

• *Counterpressure:* During contractions, applying strong and steady force to the lower back with a fist or the heel of the hand can provide a laboring woman with welcome relief. Or someone may apply pressure on both sides of the hips. It's only useful if it feels good to you, the woman who is making the effort, so be sure to communicate.

• *Hot and cold applications:* Apply superficial heat using heating pads, hot-water bottles, gel packs, warm, moist towels, and warm blankets. Apply superficial cold using ice bags, cool, moist towels, and frozen gel packs. Use whichever range of temperature feels best to you. Keep both on hand.

• *Immersion in water:* Water is very relaxing and physically supporting, as it reduces the effects of gravity on your body. Many women plan to use water to relieve pain during labor for this reason, for which they use bathtubs, whirlpools, and birth pools. Stimulation from taking a shower can also be very soothing in the midst of childbirth. Of course, using water immersion for pain management is a different matter than having a baby underwater.

• *Touch and massage:* Whether it is an affectionate pat, a hug, or a strong massage, touch communicates caring, compassion, and reassurance. Massage may involve light or firm stroking, vibrations, rolling, kneading, circular pressure, joint manipulation, or steady pressure. You must dictate your needs for more or less of a certain kind of massage you like. While acupuncture can bring pain relief, it is not practical for labor since movement is precluded while needles are inserted into the body. But acupressure, a form of massage therapy based on the same concept of energy lines and points running throughout the body, may be very useful to you.

• *Aromatherapy:* Essential oils, such as lavender, rose, chamomile, and sage, when diffused in the air, applied on a hot facecloth, or included in bath water or a foot massage, are said to produce various comforting effects. Some women are acutely sensitive to smell during pregnancy and labor, in which case these are ill advised.

• *Self-hypnosis and visualization:* When learning how to engage in self-hypnosis, you are taught how to induce a light trance state in which you perceive everything going well. This can be useful during labor. One woman went to a hypnotist–birth therapist to prepare for pain. Their session was audiotaped and she listened to the tape nightly before bed. When the time came, she says, "I don't know if it helped me. I never went into a trance state. But I certainly was well able to cope with the pain."

Similarly, successful athletes have known for years to prepare for a big game or race by visualizing how to perform effectively. This technique combines relaxation and imaging with concentration. Essentially you run the future scene over and over again in your imagination and see yourself handling different possibilities with ease and calmness. Then, when you're in the real birth scenario anything that happens feels OK. You can roll with the punches, because you've already lived through them.

• *Music and audio-analgesia:* Doula Deborah Badran told me a wonderful story of using music to avoid interventions. A woman phoned asking Deborah to attend the birth of her second child and admitted, "I'm scared to ask you to come." "Why?" Deborah asked. "It was so magical the first time, I'm afraid it won't be magical this time." With her first baby, the woman and her husband had put on big band music. At eight centimeters, they were laughing, pushing, and twirling around to Glenn Miller. They had a great time.

"Don't compare; this is a different baby," Deborah told her. Unfortunately, baby number two stalled at five centimeters and the hospital staff wanted to take the woman upstairs for interventions. Deborah suggested, "How about we do something else this time instead of dancing?" The parents got the mother rocking on her hips while singing three descending tones. As she did this, within twenty minutes her cervix had dilated fully and the baby dropped down into her pelvis. The sound opened up the woman's body and invited the baby to descend. In an hour, the baby was out.

"I have never seen this before or since," says Deborah. "Not only did the tones she and her husband sang save the woman from needing a cesarean section, the baby also came out making a similar sound to the one they were singing."

Audio-analgesia incorporates soothing sounds between contractions with white sounds (background noise) during contractions. It adds dimension and ambiance to the birth room. Although it can support rhythmic breathing and contractions, the sounds or music must be carefully chosen to appeal to the mother in labor.

• *Meditation:* Many forms of meditation exist, from silently repeating a single word or sound, known as a "mantra," to focusing on the in- and outflow of your breath. The idea is to pay attention to one thing and in the process let everything else drop away.

One overdue woman was a SCUBA enthusiast. In the hospital, her husband hung a picture—to use as a focal point—on the wall across from her bed. The picture was of the couple diving in the Caribbean with stingrays. Overnight she kept looking at it and imagining herself floating in the watery depths with her baby. Although she was supposed to get a dose of Pitocin in the morning, when the doctor checked her cervix she was almost fully dilated. He was blown away by her relaxation.

Meditation invokes deep relaxation and clarity. But it requires some practice, so you should practice it in advance of your due date.

• *Prayer:* Every religion has contemplative practices. Whether you are a Buddhist, a Christian, a Jew, a Muslim, or of any other persuasion, you've probably been taught how to pray. Spiritual people outside institutional religions also have contemplative practices. In birth, a woman must find a way to surrender to the process she's undergoing. Prayer can be appropriate in childbirth for this reason, and there are many instances in which it has helped a lot.

Kelly had such a wonderful first birth experience that she became a doula. Her second labor was very painful and a struggle. When she got pregnant with her third child everything went along well until her seventh month, when she thought her water had broken early. After she raced to the hospital and got put on a fetal monitor, she went into a panic. She had an anxiety attack due to the memory of excruciating birth pain. She says, "I had to face the fact that even after years of teaching other women about how fear makes you rigid, I couldn't overcome my own fear. I was freaking out." The only way she knew to handle her fear was to pray. "God, I don't know what to do. I need your help." It turned out she wasn't in labor and she was sent home.

Kelly, a Christian, describes, "I worried a little bit here and there up to my due date. Then on the day of labor I had such peace that I knew it wasn't from me. All of a sudden my worrying was gone. With every contraction I repeated a prayer from the Bible: 'There is no fear in love, because perfect love casts out all fear.'" By praying she was able to concentrate on staying relaxed and surrender control of the process. Then, even when the nurse had to do a maneuver toward the end of labor to change her son's position, which was stuck on a bone, she felt unafraid.

Understanding Epidurals

Once commonly given for anxiety and to enable sleep in early labor, to-day sedatives and tranquilizers are not in common use anymore. Opiates, which are stronger-acting pain medications than acetaminophen (that is, Tylenol) or ibuprofen (that is, Motrin, Advil), can be administered alone or with an epidural. A reason *not* to give these types of drugs is that they affect the body system, making a laboring woman feel groggy and sleepy. They can also cross the placenta and get to the baby.

By contrast, regional anesthesia blocks the nerves, so pain is completely shut off in the localized region of the lower body, whereas everywhere else the woman feels essentially normal. (That is, when all goes as planned.) Depending on how they're applied, these anesthetics, known as epidurals, can also cause a partial or a total motor block—meaning temporary paralysis.

What Happens When You Get an Epidural?

Let's suppose you decide to get an epidural—what actually takes place? First, your doctor, your midwife, or a labor-and-delivery nurse will give you a vaginal examination to be sure you're far enough along in labor. It's dangerous to have an epidural too soon, as the medication can stall or even stop your labor. Your baby is ready to come and you don't want to prolong labor unnecessarily. If your cervix is dilated at least five centimeters and you're progressing nicely, then there are no medical contradictions to the anesthetic.

An epidural is a highly skilled procedure involving certain risks that must be handled by an anesthesiologist. Obstetricians do not provide epidurals. Although home-birth midwives don't use epidurals, by working in concert with the anesthesiologists on staff, hospital-based midwives have the same access to epidurals for their patients that doctors do. After your vaginal exam, if it's agreed that it's OK to have one, the anesthesiologist will be called. On arrival, the anesthesiologist will talk to you about an epidural's risks and benefits. He will evaluate you, read the nurses' or midwife's notes, and/or read the EFM strips to decide for himself that you're a good candidate. If your condition appears satisfactory, you'll be asked to sign a consent form.

The spinal cord is a collection of nerves that descend from the brain down the center of the back, where nerves branch out into different areas of the body. The brain floats in a fluid that goes all the way down the spine. Just as the brain is covered, a layer of skin—the dura mater—covers the spine to hold in the cerebrospinal fluid. When the anesthesiologist injects an epidural into your body, he is not injecting it into the dura mater or into the nerves, but rather he goes through the dura mater and injects it into the fluid inside the dura. You must be properly positioned so the drug cannot move to where it shouldn't go.

So the next step, after your consent, is for the anesthesiologist to place you in the correct position for the insertion of a long needle. This position varies according to the individual practitioner. It might be leaning forward. It might be on your side. The skin on your back will be sterilized and you'll be given a little Novocain to numb your skin. You will be instructed to hold still. Then a long needle will be inserted until it is determined that the tip is in the proper place. The anesthesiologist knows he's in the right place when he feels a little pop as the needle goes through the dura. Another confirmation is that he draws back on the syringe and sees clear fluid. At this point he injects anesthesia. The procedure is not very painful for you, and it is only a couple of minutes long.

From then on, you have to be careful of your position. Usually you will be resting on your back with your head elevated. That prevents the drug from flowing "upstream" toward your brain, and keeps the drug flowing "downstream" with gravity. The anesthesiologist can speed up the flow of medication, slow it down, stop it, and otherwise adjust it as desired. If you start having more pain in a little while, the doctor can come back and give you a little more medication.

Being on an epidural can seem a little like an out-of-body experience. Not only are you no longer having pain, you are no longer having any sensations that normally go along with birth. You won't feel contractions and you won't be able to feel the birth canal opening. Except in rare cases, from the time you're given an epidural until the baby comes out you will be on the drug. That way, if there's suddenly a big problem, you are already set up to go ahead with an instrumental birth or a cesarean section. If you have any tears or episiotomies, they can be repaired while you're numbed out. The most common way to do a cesarean is with an epidural (see chapter 7).

Once the epidural line is in, and everything is fine, you must now be monitored more closely than you would be otherwise. A sudden drop in blood pressure is a serious and common complication of epidurals, which means birth attendants have got to do something immediately. With a drop in pressure, a baby can get cut off from the blood supply, thus getting insufficient oxygen and becoming brain damaged in a matter of minutes. That's why you will be kept on an IV and an electronic fetal monitor. You could be in the bed for half an hour or for ten hours. You are having a full medical birth.

Once your baby comes out and everything is sewn up that needs to be, the anesthesiologist will remove the epidural needle from your spinal cord. Sensations will begin returning from within a few minutes to a few hours—this varies. In some cases, the effects can last longer than that. You have to be watched closely for at least a couple more hours as your blood pressure may drop.

Appropriate reasons for a caregiver to consider giving an epidural are:

• *Induced or augmented labor:* If a woman is given a drug either to kick-start or to speed up labor, her uterus will begin contracting both faster and more intensely. This can put enormous stresses on the woman's body, which otherwise would have been more gradually prepared for the act of giving birth. As a result, pain is magnified to such a degree that in many instances an epidural becomes necessary to control pain.

• *Cesarean section:* Anytime a woman has surgery she needs strong pain medication. During most cesarean sections a woman is awake and requires regional anesthesia, such as an epidural. In fact, if labor has been induced or augmented chances are that the woman is already receiving epidural medication. For the surgery, it is continued. During other types of major surgery, such as to repair a uterine rupture, it is sometimes necessary for the woman to be rendered unconscious with a general anesthetic.

• *Extreme pain:* As we saw earlier, everyone's tolerance for pain differs. Depending on the structure of a woman's body, the size of the baby, the position the baby assumes inside her body, and other issues arising in the moment, pain may feel too difficult to manage. In these cases, it may sometimes be reasonable for a woman to turn to epidural for relief.

• *Extreme exhaustion:* If the duration of the first and second stages of labor is several days, a woman's strength may falter. To achieve some necessary rest, a few hours of pain relief under the influence of an epidural can be appropriate for exhaustion.

Questionable reasons for a caregiver to consider giving an epidural:

• *Routine:* Although you will have to make the decision for yourself, based on personal knowledge of your ability to persevere and manage pain, the potential complications of having an epidural make the purely routine use of the drug unwise. I strongly recommend that you explore natural techniques for reducing anxiety and tension and gaining relief from the powerful sensations of birth, before you immediately jump on the pharmacological bandwagon. You may be surprised at what you can handle.

How Safe Is an Epidural?

As the possible recipient of an epidural, it is important for you to make up your own mind about its safety—weighing its risks against its benefits. Although women are often willing to take risks with their own bodies to gain pain relief, it is highly unlikely that a well-informed woman would be willing to put her baby at unnecessary risk. Nonetheless, that's the approach the medical community has embraced in the past decade.

In *The Thinking Woman's Guide to a Better Birth*, award-winning medical author Henci Goer says, "Many anesthesiologists, doctors, nurses, and even some midwives tend to live in a black-and-white world. They believe that labor pain has no value, mastering labor pain has no value, and epidurals have no defects. These beliefs color perception in ways that are obvious to those who don't share them but invisible to those who do."[4]

One in four women receiving epidurals experience complications.[5] Statistics show that the risks are many and often serious, starting with an increased possibility of the woman's death.[6] Complications may include puncture wounds at the insertion point near the spine, low blood pressure, nausea and vomiting, short-term backache, headaches, shivering, and prolonged labor. Rare, yet more severe problems include trouble breathing, brain damage, and death. Complications for the baby may include low blood pressure, toxicity, and fetal malposition. The list of risks below is intended to help you assess the degree of safety of epidural (low, moderate, or high) so you can make an informed choice when this option is offered to you.[7]

- *Maternal death:* The maternal mortality rate for women receiving an epidural for normal labor pain is three times higher than for women in normal labor who don't receive the block. However, the risk is low.

- *Temporary paralysis:* For every 500 epidurals performed there will be one case of temporary paralysis following the birth. Paralysis will be permanent in the case of one out of every half million women who receive an epidural.

- *Slowing things down:* A great deal of scientific research has shown that women receiving an epidural block for normal labor pain will have a significantly longer second stage of labor. This, in turn, results in a four times greater risk of using forceps or vacuum extraction, and at least a twofold greater risk of cesarean section. Of course, instrumental and surgical births carry their own serious risks, as does the anesthetic (see chapters 5 and 7).

• *Infection and fever:* A woman has a 15 to 20 percent chance of developing a fever after an epidural, necessitating a diagnostic evaluation for possible infection in both her and her baby. Evaluations can sometimes be invasive, such as those requiring a spinal tap on the baby.

• *Urinary retention:* Between 15 and 35 percent of women given an epidural will suffer from urinary retention after the birth. It usually goes away in a few hours.

• *Severe back pain:* Thirty to forty percent of women receiving an epidural during labor will have severe back pain after the birth. These may last for days or for several weeks. Twenty percent still experience severe back pain a year later.

How effective is an epidural block in relieving pain? In approximately 10 percent of epidurals it doesn't work, and there is no pain relief. Even when it works, around a third of the women given an epidural in retrospect would surely trade a few hours of pain-free labor for days or weeks of pain after the birth.[8] You may be told something on the order that recent innovations, such as changing the type of drugs used or the potency of the doses used, or using the so-called walking epidural, eliminate the risks to a laboring woman and her baby. In fact, they do not.[9]

How safe is epidural for the baby?

• *Oxygen deprivation:* A common complication of an epidural is a sudden loss of maternal blood pressure, leading to a sharp drop in blood flow through the placenta to the fetus. In 8 to 12 percent of such cases, this results in mild to severe oxygen deficiency for the fetus, as demonstrated on a fetal heart-rate monitor. Unfortunately, even when doctors try to prevent this drop in blood pressure by giving a laboring woman a big dose of fluid through an IV, it doesn't always work. So lack of oxygen is a possibility. A few studies have suggested that an infant whose mother had an epidural is more likely to show poor neurological function at one month of age.

• *Fetal malposition:* There is also a greater likelihood of fetal malposition during labor when a woman has an epidural. Her natural mechanisms for rotating the baby are interfered with because she loses normal sensation—she no longer adjusts the position of her body.

Valuable Questions

After you consider all the information on the pros and cons of the various drug and nondrug possibilities that are available to you, it is important to decide which kind of pain management you want to use during labor. Ask your care providers the following questions. Try using a few key questions you already know the answer to, so you can test their level of knowledge and willingness to tell you the truth, such as: "Does having an epidural increase the chance that I will be paralyzed?" (Correct answer: yes.)

• Why are you suggesting an epidural?

• What are the medical indications for it?

• Are there special considerations related to my specific condition?

• What is the scientific evidence that an epidural will make things better?

• What is the scientific evidence that an epidural will make things worse?

• What are the risks to me?

• What are the short-term consequences?

• What are the long-term consequences?

• Is my labor likely to be prolonged or stall with an epidural?

- How often do your patients need instrumental births after an epidural?

- How often do your patients need a cesarean section after an epidural?

- What are the risks to my baby of my having an epidural?

- What are other possible pain-relieving solutions?

- What are the risks and benefits of those alternate solutions?

- What do you see happening if the epidural is not done?

I believe that many women agree without hesitation to having epidurals—or request an epidural—because they're not being told the scientific facts about the risks of using drugs for normal, healthy labor. Indeed, at a meeting of obstetric anesthesiologists in the United States a few years ago, discussions were openly held on how to prevent information on the risks of epidurals from reaching the public. Many doctors worried that the information on risks might scare women and therefore they shouldn't be told.[10]

It is *absolutely essential* for anyone being offered an epidural to know all the scientific facts before giving informed consent to the procedure. If you understand the facts and still want or need an epidural, that's your business—a different matter altogether. I support your right to manage pain however you see fit.

Adding Your Wishes to Your Birth Plan

Labor pain and the choice of pain management is a highly personal decision. No sane person wants to suffer, no compassionate caregiver wants you to suffer, and the flawed medieval notion that labor pain is a punishment for Eve's behavior has been discarded. A significant opening and passage will occur in your body during childbirth and this may produce strong sensations. The good news is that these are temporary and your body is built for it. Like the issue of using technology and drugs to manage the stages of labor in nonemergency conditions, adding interventions to the mix can influence events—sometimes for better, sometimes for worse. Please think through the matter carefully.

Write about your hopes and fears for childbirth in your journal. What experiences of physical pain have you had in your lifetime? Have you ever been traumatized? Are you hoping to have a rich, sensual experience of birth? Does birth mean more to you than just going home with a baby in your arms? What additional meaning does it have? I suggest that you give yourself plenty of time before the birth to investigate strategies for pain management, as some methods, like self-hypnosis, have high success rates, but could take regular practice for several weeks to become effective.

If you are sure now you want an epidural, take this opportunity to discuss it with your physician. Perhaps there is a way of monitoring your desire for pain medication in the midst of the labor process that your doctor knows that would lessen your and your baby's exposure to medication. If there is anything you have learned while reading this chapter that makes you want to reassess earlier decisions, go back and review them.

We cannot discuss childbirth in America without taking a good hard look at cesarean section and episiotomy, if for no other reason than that nearly a third of the births in our nation are now surgical births. Cesarean rates are increasing and episiotomy rates are dropping. What's going on? Find out in the next chapter.

Eight

How to Know When You Need Surgery

Cesarean Section and Episiotomy

When Sandy got pregnant for the first time, she read many books and determined that, for her baby's sake, she wanted a natural, drug-free childbirth. But, as she'd never experienced the sensation of a contraction, she still embraced the possibility that in the middle of labor she might want pain relief. Although the idea of home birth was appealing, she'd never known anyone who'd given birth that way. Thus, after weighing her options, she decided to give birth in a hospital attended by an obstetrician and a doula. She was grateful that her insurance company would cover the cost of both.

Part of Sandy's detailed birth plan was to remain at home as long as possible before going to the hospital so she could walk around and rock in a rocking chair. Her biggest concern was that she'd tense up under the unfamiliar conditions at the hospital, "fail to progress" sufficiently, and end up going through a cesarean section. She wanted to maintain control of the birth scene and enjoy the experience.

The entire day before she went into labor Sandy was having frequent Braxton Hicks contractions. Such preliminary contractions are unrelated to cervical dilation and they aren't regular enough to be meaningful. Her water broke at 2:30 A.M. By 5 A.M. her contractions had grown longer and more regular, so she and her husband decided to go to the hospital. She called her doula, a good friend, who met them in the hospital room as the couple was settling in. The room had a rocking chair, so Sandy continued rocking and breathing through her contractions. It felt good.

When a nurse came to check Sandy's cervix at 6:30 A.M., she told her, "You're at seven centimeters." That was good news. "But you know what?" the nurse added. "I think I'm feeling your baby's butt, not her head." This indicated a breech, or reversed birth position, implying there would be a more difficult transition. The nurse immediately left the room, and then a series of other hospital staff came in and checked Sandy in turns. They did an ultrasound scan of her abdomen that confirmed the baby's position as feet first. By now, she was having contractions every two to three minutes and felt somewhat concerned. The time passed in a blur.

Sandy's doctor, on the way to the hospital, called her. She soothingly assured Sandy, "Don't worry, you'll be holding your baby in an hour. We're going to do a cesarean section." There was no active decision-making on Sandy's part. Cesarean section was presented to her as a done deal: necessary and hassle free. At 7 A.M., the anesthesiologist came in to explain the risks of anesthesia. Sandy's contractions were coming once a minute and they hurt. Part of her wanted pain relief, but she also wanted her baby girl to be born alert, without drugs in her system.

The staff moved Sandy to the operating room and the doctor greeted her there. Her laboring was still intense. As the anesthesiologist asked her to lean forward and prepared to give her a spinal block, Sandy said, "Wait. I'm having a contraction!" It was so clear to her that the baby was coming, since it was two full hours since she'd been at seven centimeters and this contraction felt stronger. In that moment she thought, "I could do this. I could have done it!" She looked at the clock and it was exactly 8 A.M. Everyone in the room continued with the cesarean. After only a few minutes, her daughter was born at 8:12 A.M. Sandy didn't feel anything during the surgery, except a little pressure. Then her doctor lifted the baby up, saying, "She's sure got a beautiful little tushie."

Sandy's main regret was that the anesthesia interfered with her ability to hold her baby in the operating room. She felt so groggy she could barely lift her arms. All she wanted was to sleep, and she did for a few hours. Then, she nursed her daughter in her hospital room and the two of them bonded. It was four days before she went home. It was several months until she was entirely pain free. It was a few years before the numbness of her incision scar was gone.

Although it was not the plan she'd made for the birth, Sandy was glad that her daughter was born healthy and whole. Nonetheless, she holds on to her memory of the last big contraction and wonders: Did it have to be that way? She was never told that, in fact, breech presentation is not an emergency and that the latest research shows a vaginal breech birth is as safe as a cesarean section.

The best time to plan for an emergency is before there is an emergency. Your birth plan should include everything that might happen during labor, including the possibility of cesarean section or episiotomy. This chapter will provide you with the knowledge you need to begin to evaluate your medical options if a cesarean section or episiotomy is suggested. It may also help you overcome any disappointment—to feel fulfilled—if ultimately you do require surgery and are unable to experience a vaginal birth or the birth scene you originally anticipated. Certainly, you must consider a number of factors when making decisions, including your unique circumstances, values, and emotions, as well as those of your spouse or partner.

What Happens During a Cesarean Section?

A cesarean section is the surgical term for the procedure of cutting a baby out of the mother's uterus, instead of the infant emerging through the vaginal canal. It is major abdominal surgery that when indicated can be lifesaving.

Let's suppose that you and your caregivers agree that you need a cesarean section. After this decision is made, you're wheeled on a gurney to an operating room that's specifically equipped for this purpose, where the surgical team meets you. In most cases, operating teams include two surgeons (one to perform the surgery and one to assist, kind of like a pilot and copilot of an airplane), an anesthesiologist or a specially trained nurse-anesthetist, two surgical nurses to assist, and a circulating nurse to run and fetch supplies. A pediatric nurse is present to receive and tend to the baby. And if the baby's condition is questionable because of indications of fetal distress, a neonatologist is on hand, too.

Quite often, someone is permitted to accompany you for emotional support—a husband or partner, a relation, or a doula, for example—although some hospitals frown on this, worrying that a layperson could faint during the surgery. In my opinion, it's worth insisting upon having that support there.

The steps of a cesarean are as follows. The skin of your abdomen is shaved and sterilized. Once the doctors and nurses are scrubbed in, you are anesthetized, usually with an epidural—so you remain awake. You would probably be knocked out in the case of a severe emergency, such as a uterine rupture. The anesthesiologist, in addition to administering the anesthetic, is responsible for monitoring your blood pressure, pulse, breath, lungs, and making sure you are OK. It takes approximately five minutes for the anesthetic to take effect, after which you don't feel any sensations below the waist (see chapter 7 for more on epidurals).

A screen is situated between your face and your abdomen so that you won't be able to watch the surgery. From this point on, the surgeons are completely focused on the task at hand and are unlikely to speak to you until it's over. First, they make an incision through your skin, then your muscles, then the covering of your abdominal cavity and finally your uterus. They then lift out the baby through the incision in the uterus and cut the umbilical cord. The baby is handed to the pediatric nurse. Before the surgeons close up your wounds, they remove the placenta and ensure that you are not bleeding. If they do find a "bleeder," they clamp it off to stop the flow, and then stitch it up. To finish the surgery, they suture, or sew up with dissolving threads, every layer and incision they've cut.

Due to the anesthetic, at this point, you are likely to feel very groggy. The surgeons or nurses may bring the baby over to show you and your mate or companion, but chances are you'll only get a quick look. Once the baby is born, it is taken to a prewarmed table where the nurse cleans it, checks its condition, and assigns it an Apgar score (see chapter 2). If your baby is fine, it is usually whisked away to the nursery. If your baby is not breathing or its heart is not beating properly, the nurse and the neonatologist work to resuscitate it, and instead of the nursery they take your baby to the neonatal intensive care unit, or NICU. There your baby can receive special care.

If you believe your childbirth is going to be high risk, perhaps due to preeclampsia or another serious medical condition, plan ahead. It is good to ensure that the hospital you and your doctor choose has a NICU. If there is an unanticipated emergency and your baby is born by cesarean in a smaller hospital or a community hospital that doesn't have a NICU, your baby may need to be transferred to a different hospital that does have a NICU, whereas you'll go into recovery and remain in the same hospital you gave birth. That means you'll be separated from your baby for at least a few days.

Let's assume your baby is fine after the cesarean and has been sent to the nursery. Because you've had surgery, you need time to recover. In a few hours, the epidural wears off and you begin to feel pain. Acute pain lasts for only a couple of days, whereas chronic pain from the surgery is liable to last for weeks, months, or even years. But you receive pain medication and are able to begin nursing your baby as soon as the anesthetic is out of your system (see chapter 11). If there are no complications from the surgery, you may expect to stay in the hospital for three or four days. If you are bleeding or develop an infection, your stay could be extended. Postcesarean hospital stays vary in length. A woman who undergoes cesarean due to a severe condition, such as uterine rupture, can expect a longer recovery period since her body has been through an even greater trauma.

After you and your new baby go home, you will need assistance in lifting and reaching toward objects and driving a car until your incisions are fully healed. Your surgeon monitors the progress of your healing at checkups. In approximately six weeks, for the most part you should be back to normal, ready and fully able to tend your baby.

When Is a Cesarean Necessary?

Around 5 to 10 percent of births develop serious medical complications that threaten the lives of laboring women and their babies. An obstetrician is absolutely required for such cases, as cesarean section and other invasive procedures may become a necessity.

Today, more than one million cesarean sections are done in America every year, meaning that 29 percent of births now involve this form of major abdominal surgery. According to the CDC, births by cesarean increased in 2004 for the eighth consecutive year. In 2004, the already high cesarean rate for first-time pregnancies jumped 5 percent and the rate of vaginal birth after a previous cesarean (VBAC) fell by 20 percent.[1]

During a conference in 1985 attended by sixty-two participants from more than twenty countries, the WHO, after carefully examining the scientific evidence, established an optimal rate of cesarean section of 10 to 15 percent. Ten percent is the maximum rate for hospitals that serve the general population. Fifteen percent is the maximum rate for hospitals that handle high-risk cases. In 2005, these numbers were confirmed in a global study that showed that if the rate of cesarean is significantly above 15 percent the outcomes for mothers and babies are worse.[2] Anything above those levels demonstrates that hospital staff—or some of the doctors who work there—are performing more surgery than circumstances generally warrant.

There is plenty of time for conversation with your doctor or midwife about the pros and cons of various procedures that are being recommended to you, including cesarean section. The maternity ward of a hospital is not an emergency room. So you *can* weigh your options.

Many cesareans are justifiably performed in order to save the lives of women and babies when they're in distress, but unfortunately, too many other cesareans are done unnecessarily—today more than twice as many are done in the United States than are necessary.

Appropriate reasons for which a doctor considers doing a cesarean section include the following:

- *Too fast or too slow fetal heart rate:* Both fast and slow heart rates indicate possible fetal distress. Your baby's heart may be racing more than normal because of severe stress in the process of birth. Or your baby's heart may be slowing because of oxygen deprivation. While heart rates normally increase and decrease at intervals during childbirth, especially during and following contractions, prolonged or severe changes can be an issue. Then, a cesarean section may be advisable. But the interpretation of the baby's heart rate on the electronic monitor requires careful assessment, as often it may be interpreted as showing fetal distress when there is, in fact, no fetal distress. If your midwife, nurse, or doctor interprets the monitor tracing as abnormal, he or she should always get another opinion before taking action.

- *Complete placenta previa:* At term, the placenta is covering the cervical opening.

- *Abrupted placenta:* Placenta detaches from the uterus.

- *Transverse lie:* Baby is sideways, neither headfirst nor breech, and cannot be turned.

- *Prolapsed cord:* The umbilical cord is compressed between the baby and the birth canal, and cannot be freed.

- *Hyperstimulated uterus:* Whenever the uterus contracts too rapidly, as it may if you are given a drug or an herb to "kick-start" or speed up your labor, there's less of a window between contractions for blood to flow through the placenta to your baby. Each contraction acts like a clamp on a hose. As a result, your baby may not receive enough oxygen. As we saw in chapter 6, this is an important reason to be cautious about the use of stimulants. While hyperstimulation is not a black-and-white reason to decide on a cesarean—it's a tricky indication—it increases the risk of fetal brain damage and maternal hemorrhage. After careful assessment of the monitor strip and getting a second opinion, sometimes cesarean section becomes necessary. Use the valuable questions at the end of this chapter for guidance in conversing with your caregivers.

• *Uterine rupture:* If your doctor or midwife says there are signs or symptoms of uterine rupture, you won't have time for conversation. You need an emergency cesarean. Imagine an inner tube of a tire that's burst open. This is what a uterine rupture is like. It is extremely dangerous for both mother and baby, because the baby, placenta, and blood may extrude into the mother's abdomen. Although uterine ruptures are rare, when they happen they are potentially life threatening and immediate action is required.

• *Preeclampsia:* As we discussed in chapter 6, preeclampsia can lead to complications for mother and baby during childbirth. Thus, cesarean may be needed. Because the symptoms may vary, a second opinion here is a good idea.

• *Active herpes lesions:* An estimated 30 percent of the U.S. population now has genital herpes, which is highly contagious when sores are present. During vaginal childbirth, a newborn's eyes in particular can become infected. When herpes is dormant, the risk of transmission to the baby is minimized. If you have ever had an outbreak, even if you are currently symptom free, you'll need to discuss your condition with your doctor or midwife and be prepared for the option of cesarean section.

• *Preventing HIV transmission:* Evidence shows that the rate of transmission of HIV from mother to baby is reduced by having a surgical birth. Therefore, if you know that you are HIV positive, receiving prenatal care is critical and you must be prepared for the option of cesarean. Please discuss your condition with your doctor or midwife.

Questionable reasons (often invalid) for a doctor to consider doing a cesarean section include the following:

• *The baby is "overdue":* This indication is more and more overused. Remember, half of all babies are born later than their anticipated due dates. While women often know the exact dates they conceived, usually the planned "due date" is determined by taking the date of the woman's last menstrual period, adding seven days, and subtracting three months. Forty weeks is the average length of gestation. In reality, only 5 percent of babies are born on their due date. It is perfectly normal to give birth two weeks before that date or two weeks after that date.

   If you can feel the baby kicking in your womb and there are no signs that your health is suffering or your baby is in distress, being "overdue" is not cause for alarm—just a nuisance. While doctors are more likely to want to induce labor at this point than to schedule a cesarean section (also see chapter 6), the evidence doesn't indicate that either intervention is mandated.[3] It's better to wait it out and let nature take its course, unless your pregnancy lasts beyond forty-two weeks and/or there are signs that your baby is in distress.

• *The baby is too big:* The size of the baby rarely is a significant issue. True, a fourteen-pound baby could possibly be too large to emerge naturally. But in most cases when a baby seems "stuck" in the birth canal, the baby isn't really hopelessly stuck, and it is not weight that's impeding progress. Rather it's another scenario, like the fetus is facing the wrong way. If some intervention is suggested because the baby may be too large, be sure to ask for a second opinion and confirmation of the size of the baby.

• *The baby in breech (feetfirst) position:* Childbirth generally goes more smoothly if a baby rotates inside the womb into a head-down position before pushing starts. However, for centuries midwives and doctors have been welcoming babies into the world the opposite way—feet or butt first. As long as signs of possible fetal distress are being watched for, the breech position is not an automatic signal to head for the operating room.

• *Multiple births:* Caregivers often recommend cesarean section when a woman is giving birth to three or more babies. For a twin birth the procedure is not routinely necessary, although it can be a more complicated process than giving birth to a single baby. Multiple births are more challenging situations, so please discuss your condition with your doctor or midwife, and carefully weigh the benefits and risks that both vaginal birth and cesarean section might pose to you and your babies.

• *Fibroids:* Fibroids are benign (noncancerous) tumors that grow on or within the muscle tissue of the uterus. Fibroids may be small (nut size) or large (cantaloupe size) and can occur singly or in clusters. Most do not interfere with birth, unless they block the cervical opening.

• *Diabetes:* Being diabetic is not sufficient reason alone to undergo a cesarean. However, diabetes is a risk factor during pregnancy and birth that needs to be monitored for the safety of mother and child. (See chapter 9.)

• *Obesity:* Being a large woman is also not sufficient reason to undergo a cesarean. However, if your blood pressure is high or you have another type of weight-related health condition, such as diabetes, your doctor or midwife should monitor you to determine that the labor is progressing satisfactorily and your own medical condition is under control.

• *Watching the clock:* "Failure to progress" is not a meaningful reason to intervene in the second stage of labor, although it is one that's frequently cited. The duration of labor varies widely, and policies about timing are arbitrary.

- *Preventing damage to the pelvic floor:* Some obstetricians believe that vaginal birth increases the risk of incontinence (leaking urine or feces) later on in life. Research shows that the kind of damage that leads to these problems actually relates not to normal, unforced vaginal birth, but more to the practices used during the pushing phase of childbirth, including episiotomies, forceps, vacuum extraction, and vigorous pressing on the abdomen.[4] Unless you have already suffered previous damage to your pelvic floor, a cesarean is not indicated as a preventive strategy.

- *Previous cesarean section:* VBAC is a controversial issue. A lot of doctors do repeat cesareans automatically because of their concerns about an increased risk of uterine rupture due to the scars from previous surgery. Nonetheless, if you desire to give birth vaginally, having had a previous cesarean section is not an absolute rationale for undergoing another one. Successful VBAC is possible.[5] Later in the chapter we will address the matter in greater depth.

     Although your uterus is now like a patched tire, it can hold firm. If you cannot find an obstetrician who will agree to participate, you may need to seek a midwife for assistance. Just ensure that she has a good relationship with a hospital and an obstetrician she can consult with and refer you to, if it becomes necessary. It is vital that you educate yourself and take certain precautions (see pages 148–149); still there is a good chance you can have a safe VBAC if you choose.

- *Elective cesarean:* A number of obstetricians now urge women who have no medical problems to choose cesarean section, claiming it is a woman's right to opt for any kind of birth she wants. But elective cesarean is ill considered. Like any other form of major abdominal surgery, a cesarean section has significant immediate and long-term physical risks for both mother and child. You avoid these risks by declining surgery.

Remember, if you avoid the routine use of medical interventions (see chapters 5 and 6), you can lower your chances of needing a cesarean section. Using powerful drugs to induce (kick-start) labor or augment labor (push it along) increases pain and often leads to the use of an epidural, which can slow the progress of labor and result in the need for a cesarean.

Doing a cesarean has many advantages for the obstetrician—convenience, saving time—but is there a positive side to having a cesarean for the woman in a nonemergency situation? This is tricky, because some obstetricians will promote or encourage their patients to choose a cesarean by making false claims about the procedure, such as that it's safer for the baby or will cause less damage to the mother's body. In fact, cesarean is more dangerous for the baby and causes more damage to a woman's body, both in the short term and in the long term.[6] The only real advantage for a woman to choose a nonemergency cesarean birth is the convenience of being able to schedule the time when she will have the baby.

How Safe Is Cesarean Section?

As an informed consumer, if a doctor or midwife persuaded you that a cesarean section was needed to save your life or the life of your baby, you would probably be willing to accept any risks. That's only natural. Under other circumstances, you might feel that the risks outweigh the benefits. This is a decision only you can make. But it is unlikely that you would choose to have an elective cesarean section, for instance, unless you were convinced that it was safe for you and, especially, safe for your baby.

What are the actual risks of cesarean? Are they low, moderate, or high? The list of risks below is intended to help you understand the degree of safety of cesarean so you can make a balanced judgment when the option is presented to you before or during childbirth. My intention is not to scare you unnecessarily, but rather to impress upon you some of the reasons why a cesarean is not a matter to be undertaken lightly.

- *Maternal death:* Studies show the risk of maternal death due to cesarean surgery is very low.[7] However, a woman choosing an *elective* cesarean has an almost threefold greater chance that she will die than if she gives birth vaginally. This data is based on a review of more than 150,000 elective cesarean sections.[8] Since half a million non-emergency cesareans are done every year in the United States, we can estimate that twelve American women die every year because of *unnecessary*, elective cesarean sections.

• *Hysterectomy:* There is a moderate possibility of needing an emergency hysterectomy (surgical removal of the uterus or womb) due to hemorrhage and other surgical complications either during a cesarean section or in the early weeks following a cesarean birth, leaving you infertile.

• *Side effects or accidents with anesthesia:* Regardless of why a surgical procedure is done, if anesthesia is necessary, the anesthesia itself carries a risk of death; or sudden loss of blood pressure, leading to shock; or aspiration of fluids in the mouth into the lungs. These anesthesia risks are quite low, but should not be ignored.[9]

• *Hemorrhages:* Any surgical procedure carries a risk of hemorrhage, and although the surgeon usually can control the bleeding, major abdominal surgery like cesarean section is serious business. Occasionally extremely tragic accidents happen, such as the following. A few years ago, a woman in Iowa was transferred to a university hospital during childbirth because of possible complications. At the hospital, it was decided that a cesarean section should be done. After this surgery was over and she was resting in a hospital room, the woman suddenly went into shock and died. An autopsy revealed that her obstetrician had accidentally nicked the woman's aorta, the biggest artery in the body, leading to internal hemorrhage, shock, and death. Although such dire situations are rare, as few as 1 in 10,000, with a cesarean section, as with any other major abdominal surgery, surgical and anesthesia accidents do happen more frequently, but they are usually manageable.

• *Infections:* Studies show that about 20 percent of all women who have a cesarean will experience an iatrogenic (caused by the hospital or doctor) postoperative infection.[10] This is because the hospital is full of dangerous germs to which the woman has little or no resistance. The good news is that antibiotics usually eventually control the mother's infection. The bad news is that if the woman has an infection, her newborn baby may need laboratory tests, perhaps even a spinal tap, to rule out serious infections it may have picked up.

• *Accidental extension of the uterine incision:* Once in a while, a surgeon cuts too far or the incision rips further. This can usually be sutured up; however, it means more bleeding and a bigger scar. The risk of this is low.

• *Damage to the bladder and other abdominal organs:* The surgeon may accidentally cut into the bladder or other organs, or these organs may be bruised or damaged during the procedure. While this happens only occasionally, when it does, it can lead to short- and long-term problems in the functioning of these organs.

• *Internal scarring, including adhesions:* After a cesarean section, there will always be some scarring inside the abdominal cavity. But the scars are usually small and don't cause trouble. Every once in a while (a moderate risk), something vital is scarred or scars stick together, or adhere. This can result in blockage or narrowing of the intestines, leading to chronic bowel problems, and/or to narrowing or distortion of the vagina, leading to difficult or painful sexual intercourse, which may last for weeks or months.[11]

The risks to a woman who has a cesarean do not end with that particular birth. She has less chance that she will ever be able to get pregnant again, and if she does become pregnant, there is a much greater chance that the pregnancy will occur outside her uterus—a situation that never produces a live baby and is life threatening to her. In addition, if she succeeds in carrying her next baby full term, there is an increased risk—because she now has a scar on her uterus—that the placenta, the organ that delivers oxygen and nourishment to the baby, will partially or completely detach and no longer function before her baby is born, or that her uterus will rupture. These conditions carry huge risks of brain damage or death for her baby and significant risk to her own life.

What about the risks for the baby? An emergency cesarean can save the life of a baby. But there are potential hazards. For starters, in 2 to 6 percent of all cesareans, when doctors cut open the abdomen, they cut into the baby. Even more seriously, babies born from elective cesarean section face a much higher risk of severe, acute respiratory distress syndrome in which the baby has great difficulty breathing after birth because the normal process of squeezing the fetal fluids out of the baby's lungs during passage through the birth canal has not taken place.

Another serious threat to the baby born after cesarean section, especially elective cesarean section, is that, because our estimate of when the woman has reached the end of pregnancy is often inaccurate, the cesarean section will be done too soon and the baby will be premature. This is one of the reasons why as the number of cesarean births goes up in the United States so does the number of premature babies born—and being born too early increases the risks of neurological damage and death.[12]

Both respiratory distress syndrome and being premature are major killers of newborns.[13] Of course these risks diminish when doctors wait for women to start labor spontaneously before doing the cesarean.

You have the right to refuse medical treatment even if your doctor believes it is warranted. Doctors are not permitted to do procedures that their patients have explicitly refused. So feel free to ask for as much information as you need before making a decision. And remember, the notion that cesarean section is always the surest approach is not true. It's good to carefully assess the need for undergoing a cesarean section, so that you don't unnecessarily put yourself and your baby at risk.

Valuable Questions When Considering
a Cesarean Section

As you've seen in previous chapters, no matter what procedure is being offered to you before or during childbirth, it is advisable to ask a series of questions before consenting to it. Questions usually serve more than one purpose. In the case of a cesarean, they help you to get the evidence-based information you need to make good decisions. They also give you an opportunity to remind your doctor about the wishes you've expressed in your birth plan. And they slow down the rate of unnecessary interventions.

Presuming you have chosen a doctor or midwife whose attitudes are compatible with your own (see chapter 4), I recommend the following questions. When you have an advocate with you, such as a doula or spouse, or other family member or friend, this individual may ask on your behalf, help you interpret the responses, and support you in decision-making.

- Why do you want to do a cesarean? (Always the most important question.)

- What are the medical indications for a cesarean?

- Are there special considerations related to my specific condition?

- What is the scientific evidence (chance) that a cesarean will make things better?

- What is the scientific evidence (chance) that a cesarean will make things worse?

- What are the risks to me of a cesarean?

- What are the risks to my baby of a cesarean?

- What are the long-term consequences?

Many women grieve and/or feel depressed after undergoing cesarean sections, especially unexpected ones. Even when a woman goes home with a healthy baby, the process of her pregnancy doesn't always end there. Lucy planned a home birth and ended up needing to go to the hospital for a cesarean. As she says, "I actively grieved for weeks, because I had prepared myself for a particular kind of birth and, as much as I knew to be flexible, I had the opposite experience. For my baby's benefit, I wanted a soft, sacred birth. As a woman, I also wanted to feel what it would be like to have a baby come out of my vagina. Instead, every intervention in the book was done. Although I understand that the surgery saved my baby's life, I was angry and sad because in my heart I felt cheated."

To overcome feelings of grief, anger, or shame after having a cesarean section, there are several actions you may take. First, speak with your doctor or midwife and ask for a referral to a local support group of new mothers who have undergone similar birth experiences. Give yourself permission to feel your feelings freely, and make time to feel rather than suppress them. Get physical assistance while your body is in recovery. Join the International Cesarean Awareness Network's online support group or one of their local chapters (see Resources). Talking about your emotions and listening to others are proven healing strategies.

- What are the short-term consequences?

- What are other possible solutions to this problem, including waiting longer?

- What are the risks and benefits of those alternate solutions?

- Why do you believe that doing a cesarean has a better chance of success than not having a cesarean?

- What do you see happening to my baby and/or me if the cesarean is not done?

• Is it possible to get a second opinion from another doctor or midwife on your suggestion?

If you don't understand the answers you receive, go ahead and ask for further explanation. If you don't like the answers you get or sense that your caregiver is not being 100 percent forthcoming, you are within your rights to ask for a second opinion.

Get a Second Opinion

A second opinion is *always* a good idea when cesarean section is being discussed, even in cases when a caregiver seems reasonable and responsive, and you feel you have a good working relationship. You can explain to your doctor that you believe "two heads are better than one," especially when it comes to such an important decision. You might say, "Doctor, this is not a vote of 'no confidence'—I have all the confidence in the world in you. But this is my body and I am facing a big decision. I want to leave no stone unturned in the care of my baby and me. A second doctor may have a good idea."

If you're having a hospital birth and your doctor recommends a cesarean for a questionable reason, requesting a second opinion is a powerful deterrent against abuse. If you want a truly independent second opinion you will need to go outside your doctor's circle of colleagues. After all, it is only human nature to support one's friends and professional allies.

However, we should distinguish between different kinds of cases when a doctor might suggest a cesarean. With elective surgery, you can easily get a second independent opinion because you have plenty of time. If you are in labor and the doctor recommends a cesarean and there is no immediate threat, you have some time for a second opinion. In this instance, you could call upon a doctor you have previously identified for this purpose. A true emergency situation may be the only time when a second opinion is not feasible.

When you're having an out-of-hospital birth or a planned home birth and your midwife recommends going to the hospital for a cesarean, her presence and guidance should continue once you arrive and are important in assessing the doctor's subsequent recommendations. Midwives most often are affiliated with woman-friendly doctors.

Creative Ways to Avoid a Cesarean

One effective way to decrease the chance that you will need a cesarean is to choose the right caregiver. Good scientific research proves that choosing a midwife always lowers the risk that a woman needs a cesarean.[14] If you choose a doctor who has a lower rate of doing cesareans, this is also an effective planning strategy.

Doula Deborah Badran tells her clients while they're writing their birth plans, "When you need a surgical procedure, you need one. But as long as the baby is doing OK inside the womb, which you can tell with a fetal monitor, it is preferable to exhaust your other resources. I've seen enough to know there's often a little wiggle room." She looks for creative ways to avoid a cesarean.

In one incidence, the baby's heart rate wasn't great. As the nurses were wheeling the mother down the hallway toward the operating room, Deborah asked, "Could we try one more thing? It looks as though the baby might be pressing on its own umbilical cord. Let's get Mom on her hands and knees." They flipped her client over. "The minute my client shifted her position, the whole 'tracing' nonsense stopped on the fetal monitor. Her baby was fine. We wheeled the mother back to the labor room on her hands and knees, and she stayed in that position for the duration of labor. She didn't need a cesarean."

"You have to believe in people and the outcome," Deborah wisely advises. "If a mom gets the message that it's not possible to give birth vaginally, it won't be. On some level, she'll give up. If she gets a positive message, then she stands a fighting chance."

There is a hands-on-the-belly technique to safely turn a breech baby inside the womb into a headfirst position (called external cephalic version) when you reach "term" (the thirty-seventh week of pregnancy).[15] But it is wisest to find a caregiver who knows the skill and has prior experience to do it.

Review the helpful laboring postures section in chapter 2, "Best-Case Scenario: The Stages of Healthy Labor," for various alternatives, such as birth balls, squatting, rocking chairs, and toilet sitting (see pages 32–33). Being upright, walking around, or lying on your side is considerably more effective than lying on your back.

As you learned in the preceding chapters, your choices of birth location and birth attendant can lower your risk for the interventions known to increase the possibility of ultimately requiring a cesarean section. Such interventions include having your bag of waters purposefully broken by a birth attendant before or in early labor (artificial rupture of the membranes), using drugs to induce or augment labor, and epidurals.

Vaginal Birth After Cesarean

It is standard procedure for every doctor or midwife who is working with a woman who has had a previous cesarean section to request to see her old hospital records, especially if she wants to have a VBAC. The records contain the original surgeon's notes on whether the incision made during her cesarean section was horizontal or vertical and stipulates its length. Depending on what is learned, a cesarean section may or may not be recommended as the safest alternative.

Any kind of scar, including scars from cesarean sections, can be considered a weakness on the wall of the uterus. However, if your surgeon cuts the cesarean section incision horizontally—from side to side—when the wound heals it usually heals in a more secure way than it does if the incision is cut vertically—up and down. The older, outdated way of doing cesarean sections is the vertical method. Doctors used to cut into the abdomen vertically because the uterus is pear-shaped and they thought the technique was an easier way in and, therefore, better. At the time, they didn't understand that it was a more dangerous method. Years and decades later, research proved definitely that you get a firmer-holding scar when you cut horizontally.

Obstetricians today do not do the earlier form of surgery anymore unless they are completely out of the loop of modern obstetrics and haven't kept up with the scientific evidence. Nonetheless, every so often a doctor runs across a woman who has had a vertical incision on her uterus for some reason. This informs the doctor that she is at a higher risk for uterine rupture during her subsequent pregnancy and childbirth and that she might not be a good candidate for VBAC.

Sandy, whose story of cesarean section was told earlier in this chapter, is a perfect example of an informed patient who by working with midwives was able to avoid an unnecessary second surgical birth. When she got pregnant with her second child and went to see her obstetrician, she was excited and started eagerly chatting about giving birth at home in water. She vividly remembers how the doctor raised one hand in the air and said, "Stop, Sandy. Because you had a C-section, I don't want you laboring at home." The doctor wanted to monitor Sandy closely because she felt that Sandy would be at greater risk for complications. But in doing research, Sandy learned that many complications in VBAC are connected to the use of drugs to induce or augment labor, such as Pitocin and Cytotec, which she didn't plan to allow. She decided to seek a good midwife instead and was lucky to locate one who had given birth naturally to seven children of her own.

After touring a few birthing centers, Sandy decided to give birth at home. The best of the centers she visited was farther away from the hospital than her home. Her mother would come and care for her eighteen-month-old daughter while she gave birth. The same doula would attend her. Because her first labor, except for the cesarean, had been "by the book," Sandy felt confident that her second birth could go smoothly.

When she finally went into labor one evening, however, the birth process progressed slowly. It seemed to be taking forever for her cervix to dilate. Whenever she sat down her contractions slowed or came to a halt. She walked and walked the first night, exhausting herself. Finally, at midnight, she lay down to get some sleep. She drifted, but kept being woken by her contractions. The next day passed uneventfully. As it got closer to evening the contractions started getting closer together. At 9 P.M., her birthing team returned. She was pacing around in her bathrobe, wondering why nothing seemed to be working. Her waters hadn't broken yet and the midwives told her they could do it for her, as that might speed the labor. About 4 A.M. she accepted this suggestion and got into the bathtub as she'd planned. After almost two full days of labor, she was nearly ready to give up, go to the hospital, and request a cesarean.

There's an old joke among doulas and midwives that when a woman in labor begins to curse, you can be sure the baby's on its way. Around 5 A.M., Sandy turned to her doula, sitting there holding her hand, and said, "I've got to get this [expletive deleted] baby out of me!" The doula went downstairs and informed the midwives, "She's ready to push." Sandy pushed for a few hours, falling asleep from time to time as the midwives coached her to rest and stroked her arms soothingly. As she tells it, the birth was an unbelievable experience for her. She felt completely supported. She'd sit up to hunch over and push, and when she'd lie back her attendants would have a pillow in place for her head. Between contractions, the midwives gently stretched her perineum to minimize tearing. The perineum is the area between the vaginal opening and the anus.

As the sun rose, with her husband, two midwives, and a doula alongside her, Sandy's baby was born peacefully in the water and they lifted the baby out of the water and immediately laid the baby on her chest. It was a climactic, exuberant moment, everything she and her husband had hoped it would be. The umbilical cord pulsed for several minutes, continuing to nourish the baby with oxygen. When it ceased pulsing, the midwives cut it. There were a few more contractions to expel the placenta, but she didn't find them uncomfortable. While

the water was draining from the tub, the midwives toweled the baby off and assisted Sandy to shower and dress in a clean pair of pajamas. They left Sandy, her husband, their toddler, and their newborn resting in the master bedroom, while they went downstairs to clean the kitchen and do the laundry. Her husband told her, "You look refreshed and invigorated, as though you've run a marathon."

Precautions should always be taken by a woman planning a VBAC. While a previous cesarean is not an automatic reason for a cesarean, it is nonetheless vital that you educate yourself and take the risks to yourself and your baby into consideration. If you decide to work with a midwife, it is essential that the midwife have a relationship with a hospital and an obstetrician in case of emergency. You should not attempt a VBAC if you're farther away than thirty minutes from a hospital with facilities set up for doing a cesarean and a surgeon on duty around the clock. Even if you choose to give birth vaginally in a hospital, studies have shown that it takes about thirty minutes to set up the operating room after the decision is made to do a cesarean.[16] If it is necessary, your midwife will phone ahead to the hospital and let them know to prepare for your arrival.

Make sure you constantly have a birth attendant with you while you are giving birth. VBAC is not an appropriate situation for unattended labor (see chapter 3). Having a caregiver significantly lowers the risk to you and your baby. Call your midwife or doctor at the first sign of labor, even if you might be mistaken. Once the midwife arrives, don't let her go home for lunch or leave you unattended for any other reason, even briefly. She may need to arrange backup for herself in case another client goes into labor after you.

If your previous cesarean was traumatic, you may feel frightened as the due date approaches. You may harbor lingering doubts about your body's ability to give birth vaginally and worry that interventions will again become necessary. For this reason, if you decide on a VBAC, it is important that you surround yourself with loving people who can give you encouragement, believe in the possibility of a good outcome, and respect your decision. You are more vulnerable and impressionable in the midst of labor. If people stand around holding you to a tight schedule or introduce their fears into your birthing room, you could feel pressured and tense up. Ask them for reassurance.

Plan ways to make your delivery room feel like a safe haven. Experiment with different relaxation techniques (see chapter 6). If you remain calm, your body can open up naturally, your fears can begin to diminish, and progress can be made easier.

Understanding Episiotomy

Episiotomy is a minor surgical procedure in which a doctor or midwife makes an incision of the perineum to enlarge the vaginal opening. Midwives do them much less frequently than doctors. In planned home births, episiotomies are done in around 1 percent of births; in out-of-hospital birthing centers, episiotomies typically are done in only 5 to 15 percent of births, whereas in hospitals doctors perform episiotomies in 20 to 80 percent of births they assist.[17] Unlike cesarean section surgery, this is not a lifesaving procedure.

Doctors originally believed that it was important to get the baby out as quickly as possible and that with episiotomy the baby would be born more quickly and easily. In getting babies out quickly, often forceps or a vacuum extractor was used. Making the vagina larger helped when putting these instruments around the baby's head while it is still in the vagina.

Doctors also believed that episiotomy protected women from tearing their vaginas open during childbirth. However, as long as twenty-five years ago, good research showed that episiotomy doesn't speed up childbirth and that birth should not be speeded up unless there is severe fetal distress.[18] It was also found that episiotomy *increases* the chance that the woman's vagina will tear. Unfortunately, old practices die hard. Doctors only gradually have decreased the number of episiotomies they do.

If you are giving birth and everything is progressing well, there is no truly valid reason for a caregiver to suggest an episiotomy. However, if after discussing the pros and cons with a caregiver, you are persuaded that an episiotomy is necessary, a local anesthetic is injected and the procedure takes place quickly. Of course, if you've been given an epidural you won't need that local anesthetic.

Once your baby is born and you've expelled the placenta, or afterbirth, your caregiver will swiftly clean and sew up the incision. Unless there is a complication, such as an infection, the incision should fully heal within about six weeks.

When Is Episiotomy Necessary?

Scientific evidence has proven that episiotomy is rarely necessary.[19] Appropriate reasons for a caregiver to consider doing an episiotomy:

- *Scarring or a defect on the perineum:* In order for the baby's head to fit through the vaginal opening, the perineum needs to soften and stretch. Normally, this happens without trouble arising. Scar tissue is tougher and less malleable than undamaged tissue. If any defect in this area impedes birth, an episiotomy may be required.

- *Forceps extraction:* Based on the evidence, forceps usually are not the instrument of choice in assisted childbirth (see chapter 5). If forceps are being used, however, perhaps because a vacuum extraction failed to solve the problem, an episiotomy may be necessary to make room to insert them and grasp the baby's head.

False reasons for a caregiver to consider doing an episiotomy:

- *Reduce tearing:* Episiotomies actually *increase* the possibility of tearing. Imagine that you want to divide a piece of fabric. If you try to rip it without making a cut first, isn't it much more difficult? But if you make even a tiny snip along one edge and then pull on the sides of the fabric, it easily tears. The same principle is true with your flesh. While some doctors believe an episiotomy enables them to control the extent of tearing, evidence shows they are mistaken.[20] A little tearing happens frequently and it is no big deal. Tears usually cause only minor damage to the pelvic floor, as they follow the natural "seams" of a woman's body. If necessary, they can be repaired with stitches just as easily as the lines of an incision. An episiotomy, on the other hand, cuts across all natural barriers.

- *Speed up labor:* Babies do not get stuck on the soft tissues in the vaginal opening. If a baby is not emerging, it's because it is caught on a bone rather than on the perineum.

- *Vacuum extraction:* Unless a woman has a very narrow birth canal, the extraction equipment, which measures four to five inches in diameter, easily fits into the vaginal opening and works perfectly well.

- *Prevent incontinence later in life:* Research shows that episiotomies actually *cause* the kind of damage to the pelvic floor that leads to urinary and bowel incontinence,[21] for example if the episiotomy incision extends and tears into the rectum (a fourth-degree tear). Studies clearly demonstrate that urinary incontinence correlates with giving birth to a large number of children over a lifetime, having a baby whose birth weight is more than ten pounds, having a baby pulled out with forceps or vacuum extraction, and having an episiotomy.[22] The risk of fecal incontinence is shown to increase twenty-two-fold with a midline episiotomy.[23]

How Safe Is Episiotomy?

What are the risks—low, moderate, or high—that an episiotomy will contribute to health problems during and after childbirth?

- *Tearing:* When the perineum tears a little bit, or even a lot, and the tears are confined to this area, the tearing is considered "first degree" or "second degree." The perineum is in the area that often tears naturally. "Third-degree" or "fourth-degree" tearing occurs when tears extend toward or into the rectum. The risk of first- and second-degree tears is moderate with a first baby and much less with subsequent childbirths. The risk of third- and fourth-degree tears is normally very low, but is increased by the use of episiotomy.[24]

- *Hemorrhage:* Episiotomy always increases the risk of hemorrhage. If the tear follows along the natural lines of the body, it is less likely to rip into blood vessels than an episiotomy that crosses the muscle fibers. But in either case, some damage is done to tissues and so bleeding occurs. The bleeding is usually controllable.

- *Infection:* After childbirth it is normal for fluids to seep out of the vagina, because the uterine wall is raw and healing. Until the skin around the incision is completely healed, even after it has been sutured, it is vulnerable to infection.

- *Painful urination:* Some women experience stinging sensations when they urinate after an episiotomy. But this is a short-term problem, which only lasts until the episiotomy is healed.

- *Long-term sexual problems:* If the episiotomy has extended into a severe tear, or if a surgeon does a poor job in stitching up the incision, the vagina can be deformed in one way or the other, leading to painful intercourse.

Valuable Questions When Considering Episiotomy

As always, when a caregiver suggests a procedure, it is important to ask questions. Here are some suggestions of what you might ask in order to make an informed decision.

- Why do you want to do an episiotomy?

- What are the medical indications for it?

- Are there special considerations related to my specific condition?

- What is the scientific evidence that an episiotomy will make things better?

- What is the scientific evidence that an episiotomy will make things worse?

- What are the risks to me?

- Am I more or less likely to tear with an episiotomy?

- What are the short-term consequences?

- What are the long-term consequences?

- How often do your patients hemorrhage after episiotomy?

- How often do your patients have sexual problems after episiotomy?

- How often do your patients get an infection in their episiotomy incision?

- What are other possible solutions to this problem?

- What are the risks and benefits of those alternate solutions?

- What do you see happening if the episiotomy is not done?

Avoiding Episiotomy

The most reliable way to avoid an episiotomy is to choose a birth attendant who does few of them. Then the issue is much less likely to come up. You can determine a caregiver's rate of episiotomy in the initial interview when you are selecting a doctor or midwife (see chapter 4). The next most reliable way to avoid the need for episiotomy is to refuse the suggestion to use forceps and/or vacuum extraction, unless it's absolutely necessary.

Numerous problems are created when a caregiver wants to speed up labor. The trouble with hurrying to get the baby out is that it doesn't give the mother's body the time required to expand and open safely. Skin is naturally elastic and can stretch like mad, but it cannot stretch in one second or two seconds. Stretching has to occur gradually. That's why allowing nature to take its own course prevents tearing.

One of the most important things that midwives do for a woman in childbirth that most doctors and labor-and-delivery nurses do not do is they let her take her time without continually urging her to "push, push, push." When the baby's head is crowning, it is not seen as a sign to pull the baby out. They don't try to hurry things along or rush to catch the baby. Rather, they gently massage the perineum as it slides over the baby's head. If the baby's head does not burst through the vaginal opening, the skin normally expands enough to accommodate it with a minimal amount of tearing at worst, and often none.

Adding Your Wishes to Your Birth Plan

Cesarean section is such an important contingency that I recommend creating a separate section in your birth plan covering this possibility. You'll be guided in chapter 13 on the kind of language and bullet-point issues you might choose to include. For now, let's just admit that if you are planning a vaginal birth, a VBAC included, this is going to be your backup plan—an eventuality that you do not wish to see happen, but a real lifesaver if it does. If it becomes a necessity, you'll be glad to have addressed it ahead of time.

Planning is not planning for an outcome, but for a process. Your opportunity to have a satisfactory experience of a surgical birth is to plan for the setting, the doctor, your companions/advocates, the postnatal baby care, and your recovery process. Those are under your control, as is your perspective on surgery. Your main goal is getting home safe and sound, and your surgeon, if surgery is necessary, should be seen as your ally. On a fresh page in your journal, reflect on how you would like to be helped. What would you require to be comfortable with the possibility of a cesarean?

Have conversations with your doctor or midwife about cesareans and episiotomies, based on the valuable questions listed above. Tell your caregiver how you feel, listen to his or her opinions and attitude, and make notes for your planning process. These are difficult, serious, and important matters to strategize about and mull over. It's important to let your spouse or partner and family understand your wishes in these regards.

With this discussion, we've finished evaluating all the most popular birth interventions. Another major point of concern that pregnant women need to address during their planning is whether or not they are healthy going into childbirth. What additional risks would factor into the previous scenarios we've considered? Do any need to be covered in your birth plan? Is your pregnancy high risk or low risk, and what exactly does that mean when choosing a birth location, primary attendant, and possible interventions? The next chapter covers physical, mental, and emotional risk factors in pregnancy.

Nine

Are You High Risk or Low Risk?

The Answer May Not Be What You Expect

Diana and Marco North were excited about the impending birth of their daughter and prepared in every way they could imagine for a natural birth. They attended childbirth classes together, and Diana did hundreds of Kegel exercises every day to prepare her perineum. Careful about her exposure to chemicals, she ate only organic produce, meats, and milk. At nineteen weeks, her obstetrician advised Diana to undergo a whole battery of tests, after which Diana was informed that there was a problem with her placenta: It was "lying low" and there was a possibility she would develop placenta previa, a rare high-risk condition in which the placenta partially or entirely covers the cervix. Of course, Diana felt anxious about it. She began extensively researching the placenta.

In her prenatal visit the next month, she told the doctor she had been sleepless worrying and wished she'd been given more of an explanation about her placenta. In her office, the doctor showed the Norths charts on moving placentas. The ultrasound done that day revealed "marginal placenta previa." The condition was improving. Physically, Diana had an easy, trouble-free pregnancy. With a marginal placenta previa women sometimes will bleed a little. She didn't bleed and she felt great in every way—except emotionally. Everywhere she went people kept filling her head with disaster scenarios. It was hard to know whose opinion to believe about the possible risks she faced in childbirth.

What are some of the health conditions a pregnant woman might face that dictate more or less caution as she goes into labor? What consideration should be paid to the age of the mother? What steps can be taken leading up to childbirth to counteract these risk factors? Which conditions would dictate giving birth in a hospital setting under a doctor's care? In this chapter, we'll explore the risk approach to childbirth and what it could mean for you.

What Does It Mean to Have a "High-Risk" or a "Low-Risk" Pregnancy?

As my book *Pursuing the Birth Machine* describes, the risk approach is a triage system in which a pregnant woman is screened to see if she has any of a list of risk factors, such as diabetes, high blood pressure, HIV, herpes, and so on. Depending on the presence or absence of these risk factors, the woman is placed in a low-risk or high-risk category and the care she receives will vary depending on her risk category. This applies mainly to prenatal care, which is not the central topic of this book.[1] Nevertheless, a few words about it are in order, partly because your risk status influences how the hospital staff treats you when you go to the hospital to have a baby. The idea is to screen a pregnant woman so measures can be taken to prevent complications before they arise or catch them early enough to reduce or eliminate potential harm to the woman and her baby. While this approach has advantages, it also has serious disadvantages, not the least being that it leads to quick interference in childbirth at the first sign of deviation from normal.

Interestingly, how most doctors would define "normal" and how midwives define "normal" is not the same. If you asked a doctor and a midwife: "Are breech births considered normal?" the midwife would probably say yes and the obstetrician would probably say no, as doctors typically view breech (feetfirst) presentations as pathological occurrences. Should an out-of-hospital midwife attend at the birth of twins? Midwives don't have a consensus on this—some would, some wouldn't. Obstetricians say twins mandate a hospital birth.

Of course it is appropriate that any significant medical or psychological conditions you have will influence how your care is managed during labor. But the risk approach rejects the long-held view that birth is a normal part of the life cycle and replaces it with the view that birth is a medical event requiring as much outside help as possible if there is to be any chance of a normal result. This risk approach focuses on the negative—what can go wrong—and treats pregnant women as though they have an illness and views birth as normal only in retrospect, after it has happened. Until then, all births must be considered risky.

If you find yourself worrying excessively about giving birth, it may be partly because you have embraced this interpretation. The risk approach assigns too many pregnant women to the high-risk category. As a result, many healthy women view pregnancy and childbirth as dangerous, even if they are low risk. Furthermore, being labeled at risk increases a woman's level of stress, which is not good for her or her baby and certainly doesn't facilitate labor. Remember, relaxation is the key. Women at risk need social and emotional support. If you're one of them, reach out and ask for help.

It is important for you to know that your risk situation may change. It is also very important that if you are put into a high-risk category, you carefully investigate why and, perhaps, get a second opinion. If the evaluation is fully warranted, learning what you can do to handle your risk factors may be critical to your health and the health of your baby.

Let me make one more point here before we move on to discussing individual risk factors. Midwives who attend planned out-of-hospital births specialize in providing ongoing prenatal care and labor support to low-risk women. Like obstetricians, they use professional guidelines that enable them to assess a pregnant woman's risk for various complications. If they find a problem, they either contact their supporting obstetrician or entirely turn the care of a woman over to a physician. But there is a major difference between midwives' and doctors' risk-assessment policies.

The medical approach, generally, is to prefer a medical risk to a natural risk, feeling that instruments, drugs, and surgery are under a doctor's control—or at least more so than a woman's body left to its own devices. The midwifery approach, generally, is to trust women's bodies, and not intervene unless signs of serious problems arise. Midwives aim to assess risks that preclude a woman from giving birth naturally. They spend time getting to know a woman's individual variations very well, so when her condition changes they know how much of a deviation she's truly experiencing and exhibiting. Normal is going to be a range that varies from woman to woman.

Physical Risk Factors

In risk assessment, the bottom line for doctors is excluding a long list of problems that might occur. Their focus is on diagnosis—finding something wrong—and treatment—doing something about it. The bottom line for midwives is answering the question, Is there any reason this woman cannot have a normal birth? Doctors don't always agree with other doctors about risk factors. Midwives don't always agree with other midwives about risk factors. And doctors and midwives don't always agree. However, the following conditions or situations merit attention.

Multiple Pregnancy

Multiple pregnancy—carrying twins, triplets, or more babies—is increasing in frequency due to the newer forms of infertility treatment, such as in vitro fertilization, a procedure in which more than one egg is intentionally fertilized in an effort to increase the chance of a woman getting pregnant. In 1980, 1.9 percent of all pregnancies were multiple and, by 1999, 3 percent of all pregnancies were multiple.[2]

Multiple pregnancies carry certain increased risks for anemia, hypertension, preeclampsia, and "preterm" labor (going into labor too early: more than two weeks before the expected date). Because of these risks, it is advisable for closer management during a multiple pregnancy, with more frequent prenatal visits, and if the pregnancy is being followed by a midwife, closer collaboration with a physician. Because there is a tendency in multiple pregnancies to go into labor too early, prolonged bed rest has been advocated for many years. However, careful review of the evidence does not support this view.[3]

While some doctors will want to do an elective cesarean section on every multiple pregnancy, the available evidence, which admittedly is limited, does not support this practice. There is no evidence, for instance, that scheduling a cesarean section for a multiple pregnancy reduces the chances that a baby will die.[4] Because cesarean carries significant risks for woman and baby (see chapter 8), vaginal birth remains the best option in most cases of multiple pregnancy.

Breech Birth

Breech birth is the term for when the baby in the uterus is presenting buttocks, knees, or feet toward the birth canal at the time of birth. This is not a pathological situation, but rather a variation of the usual "vertex" birth in which the baby is presenting its head to the birth canal. If the baby is lying in the uterus with feet first or bottom down during pregnancy, there is no cause for concern because, while about 15 percent assume this position in the middle of pregnancy, all but 3 to 4 percent turn to the preferred head-down position by the end of pregnancy.[5] If the baby is still in a breech presentation near the end of pregnancy, there is still the possibility for a trained midwife or doctor to turn the baby to a headfirst position by executing a certain maneuver called external cephalic version (ECV) that involves pressing the hands on the woman's abdomen. ECV has been shown to be safe and effective in sometimes turning the baby to headfirst.

Warning: If you haven't been trained, do not attempt this maneuver.

There is a slight increased risk of birth complications with a breech presentation, both because the buttocks or feet do not open the birth canal as effectively as the head does if it goes first, and because the birth attendant in a breech birth must be skilled in how to manage the passage of the baby through the birth canal. Many birth attendants these days have not had sufficient experience in assisting at a vaginal breech birth to manage it, although there are many midwives who are highly skilled at this type of birth.

There are two approaches to how to manage breech birth at the end of pregnancy: elective cesarean section and vaginal breech birth. Prior to the year 2000, the scientific evidence favored a trial of vaginal breech birth. For this purpose, it is essential to have a skilled midwife or doctor experienced in assisting at breech birth. But for many years some doctors preferred elective cesarean section for breech and promoted it. Then in 2000, the results of a large trial of cesarean breech versus vaginal breech was published, suggesting that cesarean breech is safer.[6] As the results of this trial favored cesarean section, many physicians who already preferred cesarean birth jumped on the bandwagon of limiting breech birth to cesarean section.

Gradually scientists have looked more closely at this trial and discovered serious problems with the way it was conducted. Some cases should not have been in the trial, for instance, because in the great majority of vaginal breech babies having difficulty, the problem had nothing to do with the vaginal birth but rather it had to do with the fact that too many of the doctors who were assisting at the vaginal breech births had insufficient experience with this type of birth. There were other problems, too. In January 2006, after a careful review of all the evidence, the authors of an article published in *The American Journal of Obstetrics and Gynecology*, a leading obstetric journal, concluded that the original breech trial recommendation—that cesarean breach is safer—should be withdrawn.[7] Currently, there is not an agreement on whether the evidence favors cesarean or vaginal breech birth, and both possibilities should be available to women.

If you have a breech baby at the end of pregnancy, you will need to decide for yourself between a vaginal birth and cesarean birth. In some areas today it is difficult to find hospitals where a woman is allowed to have a vaginal breech birth. So, if this is your choice—and it is a perfectly legitimate choice—you will need to find the proper caregiver and the proper hospital to have a vaginal breech birth.

Diabetes

If a woman is diabetic prior to pregnancy, she faces definite risks. Therefore her care will need to be supervised by a physician during pregnancy and childbirth in order to keep her medical condition under good control. This protects the baby, too. A diabetic woman has a greater risk of having a newborn baby that's considered much larger than normal. This is a condition called macrosomia, and it has implications for both labor and birth. Macrosomia has two definitions. It can mean a baby is estimated to weigh more than 4,000 grams, or 8 pounds 13 ounces, as 11 percent of newborns are. Or it can be defined as a baby estimated to weigh more than 4,500 grams, or 9 pounds 15 ounces, as 2 percent of newborns are.

It has been shown that if a pregnant woman's diabetes is kept under control—meaning that she has optimal blood sugar management—there is less likelihood for her baby to be huge.[8]

How can you predict macrosomia? As the end of pregnancy approaches, the size of a baby may be estimated either by a midwife or doctor manually palpating a woman's abdomen, or by using ultrasound technology. Believe it or not, studies show that estimation by a clinician is just as accurate as an ultrasound. Having a large baby per se is not a problem, yet it is a big problem (pun intended) if the baby is too big to fit through the mother's pelvic bone outlet. In a condition called *cephalopelvic disproportion*, where the baby's head is bigger than the mother's bony pelvic outlet, the baby gets stuck on its way out of the birth canal.

There are two ways to manage the process of labor and birth if it is estimated to involve macrosomia. The first way is by scheduling an elective cesarean section before labor begins or at the onset of labor. The second way is with "expectant management," an approach in which the labor is allowed to progress with vigilance for possible signs of the baby getting stuck. The scientific evidence suggests that expectant management is preferable to cesarean, as the woman's diabetes can be controlled confidently throughout labor with an appropriate IV and in the presence of skilled senior staff. There's no reason to do a cesarean section before a diabetic woman's expected due date of delivery in the case of an uncomplicated pregnancy. And induction or augmentation of the labor with drugs is contraindicated in macrosomia, as these would simply pound the baby's head against the pelvic bone.

Perhaps you have heard the phrase "gestational diabetes" in reference to elevated blood sugar (glucose) in a pregnant woman who is not normally diabetic. Formerly elevated blood sugar was thought to represent a temporary form of diabetes. For years, some doctors considered this an important condition that had to be diagnosed and treated, and they asked their pregnant patients to take a glucose tolerance test to screen for it. More recently, scientific study shows that gestational diabetes is a false condition. The diagnosis is based only on a single abnormal glucose tolerance test. But at least 50 to 70 percent of the time, if the test is repeated after a positive result, the results of the second test will measure a normal blood sugar level.[9] Therefore, it's clear that increased risks from this so-called condition have been considerably overemphasized. In addition, when women with positive test results are treated with insulin, which is the usual treatment for diabetes, no clear improvement has been found in their infants' survival rate.

Allowing your doctor or midwife to perform an isolated glucose-tolerance test on you has the potential to do you more harm than good. Once a screening process labels a woman as a diabetic her pregnancy is considered high risk. To follow up, practitioners then use the diagnosis to invoke more extensive tests and interventions of unproven benefit to either her or her child. Available scientific evidence does not support screening all pregnant women for "gestational diabetes."[10]

High Blood Pressure (Hypertension)/Preeclampsia

Any woman who has ever been pregnant knows that she's always having her blood pressure taken and her urine tested—and for good reason. Two different hypertensive disorders are common in pregnancy, and both types of elevated blood pressure can lead to negative outcomes. Chronic hypertension, which exists prior to pregnancy, is unrelated to pregnancy although it coincides with it, and it persists after birth. Pregnancy-induced hypertension (PIH) first appears in the course of pregnancy and is reversed by giving birth.

While there are no increased risks for either woman or baby in pregnancies only characterized by PIH, if elevated blood pressure is accompanied by protein in the urine, these are considered signs of preeclampsia, a serious condition that does pose increased risks for both woman and baby. Having chronic, or preexisting, hypertension is a major predisposing factor for preeclampsia. In addition, preeclampsia may have devastating consequences, including progressing into full-blown eclampsia: seizures and/or coma in the birthing woman. Elevated blood pressure and protein in the urine are symptoms of a serious underlying disorder of the woman's circulatory system. Preeclampsia requires close medical management and treatment, often with hospitalization.

These disorders of hypertension in pregnancy occur mainly, but not exclusively, in women having their first pregnancies. A diastolic blood pressure (the lower of the two figures given for every blood pressure) between 90 and 100 mmHg is considered to be a threshold between pregnant women at low risk and women at high risk of complications.

While edema, or swelling from lymphatic fluid buildup, especially of the ankles, affects 85 percent of women with preeclampsia, it is also common in pregnant women without preeclampsia, so edema should not be used as a defining sign.

Since hypertension and protein in the urine usually occur without any noticeable symptoms, they must be detected by screening. Hence the frequent testing by healthcare providers. Simple blood pressure measurements remain an integral part of care during pregnancy and birth. Since protein in the urine in a woman with PIH or preexisting hypertension is associated with a marked increase in risk for woman and baby, testing the urine with a dipstick is also a valuable screening tool.

HIV and AIDS

You could be infected with the HIV virus, which can eventually give you AIDS, without knowing it and without experiencing any symptoms. Being aware of asymptomatic HIV is important to every pregnant woman—and to all those planning to become pregnant—because there is a risk of transmitting the virus from mother to fetus or newborn infant. Transmission from mother to fetus may occur during pregnancy, at birth (when most transmissions occur), or through breast milk. Fortunately, this event is not inevitable. The possibility can be significantly reduced by proper medical treatment of the mother during pregnancy.

As all women having the HIV virus, both those who are symptomatic with AIDS and those who are asymptomatic, may transmit the infection to their infants, universal screening for HIV of all pregnant women in now widely advocated, followed by providing medical treatment during pregnancy to those with positive test results.

Genital Herpes

It is important to have your genitalia examined by a midwife, nurse, or doctor at the beginning of your labor because you could be having your first herpes outbreak at the time of giving birth, even if you've never known you had a herpes infection of your genitalia. The risk of transmission of herpes from mother to baby at the time of birth is high as the baby comes through the birth canal, especially in a woman having her first genital herpes outbreak, as first occurrences tend to be much more severe than subsequent outbreaks.

While the risk of transmission from mother to baby is lower for a woman with chronic, or recurrent, genital herpes than a woman having an initial outbreak, if you are prone to recurrent genital herpes lesions, it is important to determine if you have an active lesion at the time of birth. A herpes infection of the newborn, acquired from the mother during birth, while rare, is a potentially serious condition. And while treatment of genital herpes with the new antiviral drugs may help to reduce the chance that you'll have an active lesion when you go into labor, there is no guarantee. Therefore you still need to have your genitalia examined when labor begins.

The current recommendation is that cesarean section should be carried out if there is clinical evidence on examination of an active outbreak of genital herpes disease.

Obesity

For women who are within the normal weight range and not obese, there is no evidence that dietary restriction of any sort during pregnancy confers benefits either to them or to their offspring. Receiving proper nutrition is important for pregnant women and their developing fetuses, of course. To prevent a serious congenital defect called *neural tube defect*—a severe neurological defect in the brain and/or spinal cord of the fetus—for instance, women who expect to become pregnant should ensure an adequate intake of folic acid, at least around the time of conception, either through supplements or their eating plan.

Overweight women and especially obese women are at high risk during pregnancy and childbirth and need close monitoring and management. The overall occurrence of being overweight and obese is dramatically increasing in the United States. Today, one out of every five women of childbearing age is significantly obese.[11] When obese women become pregnant, they need to watch out for many complications, including the following:

- Having a baby with birth defects

- Hypertension and preeclampsia

- Having a fetus that is large for its gestational age

- Labor and birth complications, including longer duration of labor

- Death of the fetus and newborn infant

In one large study of 800,000 pregnant women, seriously obese women had five times as much preeclampsia, three times as many stillborn babies, four times as many overly large babies, and more than three times as many incidences of death of the newborn infant.[12] For women who were obese, but less seriously so, the risks were similar, just to a lesser degree.[13]

Fifty years ago there was a widespread belief among doctors that all women should be put on a strict diet and not gain more than twenty pounds during pregnancy. Doctors no longer hold this belief. Today the recommended total weight gain during pregnancy for a woman of normal weight is between twenty-five and thirty-five pounds. However, because of the increased risks of adverse outcomes for obese pregnant women, the recommended weight gain for an overweight pregnant woman is only fifteen to twenty-five pounds. For an obese pregnant woman weight gain should be limited to fifteen pounds.

Ask your primary healthcare provider to help you determine your body mass index if you suspect you are overweight, and let you know which of the guidelines we've just discussed is appropriate for your situation.

"Older" Pregnant and Birthing Women

Pregnant women over thirty-five used to almost automatically fall into the high-risk category. No more, although a few doctors still mistakenly believe so. Doctors' earlier anxiety about pregnant older women has subsided as increasing numbers of "older women" are having babies safely. Since the 1990s there's been an increase of 27 percent in women aged thirty-five to forty having a baby and an increase of 44 percent in women aged forty to forty-four having a baby.[14] Therefore, we now have the evidence to understand that it is a mistake to look at age alone as a risk factor. Instead, focus is placed on risks for complications such as preeclampsia, which may be slightly heightened in older women but, nonetheless, can be managed safely.

While it is true there is an increased risk of chromosomal abnormalities in women over thirty-five, these abnormalities are no longer as feared as they once were for two reasons. First, with the advent of fetal ultrasound and genetic counseling, it is possible to screen for chromosomal abnormalities and, if they turn out to be present, give the woman the option of a medical abortion. Second, although the risk for these abnormalities goes up after age thirty-five, this increasing risk must be put into perspective. Down's syndrome, the most common chromosomal abnormality, for example, is a combination of mental retardation and physical abnormalities caused by the presence of an extra chromosome in the baby. At age twenty-five, a woman has a 1 in 1,250 chance of having a child with Down's syndrome. At age thirty, the chance rises to 1 in 1,000. At age thirty-five, it is 1 in 400. And at age forty, it is 1 in 100.[15] For most women, a 1 in 100 chance is pretty good odds and worth the risk, especially if she can be screened for the problem early enough in pregnancy.

The risk of miscarriage during the first third of pregnancy is increased in women older than thirty-five, but it is still only 20 percent, or one in five.[16] After an early miscarriage, you can, of course, try again. There is also an increase in placental problems, such as placenta previa, a condition where the placenta attaches itself over the cervical opening. This problem can be identified during pregnancy, and then followed and managed if it's still present at the time of labor. As the placenta often gradually migrates out of the way, the problem may resolve itself.

While the newborns of women in their forties have slightly more complications shortly after birth, there is no higher rate of deaths among the babies of older mothers. The vast majority of babies recover and do just fine.

One risk the older pregnant woman faces is that the rate of cesarean section doubles. These added cesarean sections are almost all elective, however—planned—and not emergencies. Doctors get anxious because they see these as "premium pregnancies," meaning that the women have tried to have a baby for a long time and view this as the last opportunity to have a baby. This is ironic and also unfortunate, as the risks for both the woman and her baby are slightly greater with cesarean section than with vaginal birth.

Women thirty-five and older who are pregnant have increased risk for some complications, but the risks are modest. Most can be managed with good care during pregnancy, labor, and birth, and in the newborn period. So, if you are thirty-five or older and you want a baby, go for it. Just be sure to get good care from someone who doesn't see your age as a big problem, but rather as a small problem that can be managed—and usually without invasive technologies.

Mental and Emotional Risk Factors

A pregnant woman's mental and emotional condition is a major component of a safe and empowering birth. In the case of a woman with a diagnosed psychiatric disorder, any medications she is taking regularly must be reevaluated in light of her pregnancy. In the case of a woman with extreme anxiety and mistrust due to the trauma of earlier sexual abuse or physical battery, caregivers must behave in an enlightened and respectful manner. The more tense the woman becomes, the more likely problems such as failure to progress will arise during the labor, the less she will enjoy giving birth, and the harder it will be for her to bond appropriately with her baby afterward.

Psychiatric Disorders

Our knowledge of the risks to the fetus of antidepressants, mood stabilizers, antianxiety drugs, and psychotropic drugs taken by a pregnant woman is incomplete. However, all these substances can pass through the placenta to the fetus, and the FDA has approved none for use during pregnancy. The data that exists suggests the possibility that the use of psychiatric drugs could increase the risk to a woman's fetus of congenital malformations. On the other hand, discontinuation of such medications carries a significant risk for relapse of the psychiatric symptoms they are supposed to be treating. Thus, a pregnant woman with the support of her caregivers is faced with a difficult personal decision in regard to the use of psychiatric medications. If you have this situation, you will need to consult with your personal physician and possibly also a psychiatrist knowledgeable about psychiatric medication in pregnancy.

Survivors of Sexual Abuse, Including Rape

Survivors of sexual abuse are at risk during childbirth, as they can have special symptoms and require special care. Studies of these women reveal a mistrust of their own bodies, a mistrust of caregivers, a fear of pain, phobias of vaginal exams and other invasive procedures, and a near-universal general fear of losing control during childbirth.

As one woman commented on an Internet chat room for survivors of sexual abuse, "The less I am 'messed up with' during the childbirth, the better I do. Anytime the control is taken out of my hands and put into the hands of a medical professional, it brings back the terror and the powerlessness of the abuse all over again."

All of these feelings may lead to refusing examinations, especially vaginal exams, which can feel like a repeat of the abuse. And often the feeling of loss of control leads to the woman's unconscious holding up the labor when it reaches a certain point, most often in the first stage, leading to labor dystocia, or failure to progress in labor. This failure to progress is best dealt with not with drugs to stimulate labor, but by using time, patience, and continuing encouragement from the woman's support team. Routines can easily be altered. For example, vaginal exams can be dispensed with, as a skilled birth attendant has no difficulty judging the progress of labor using other signs.

According to estimates, at least one out of every four American women has been molested in childhood.[17] On a subconscious level, these women and women who have been raped often fear birth and perceive it as a new violation. It is an honest and understandable reaction for such a woman not to feel comfortable with the hand of a male doctor inside her vagina, or not to feel comfortable when she is bearing down during contractions. One doula gives all the women she attends the same encouraging speech in case she is talking to a survivor of abuse who doesn't want to talk openly about it. She says, "Some of the elements of childbirth may be similar to abuse, but there are additional elements involved. And at the end, you get a present: your baby."

If a survivor tells her directly about abuse, she reminds them, "This is your day and the perpetrator of your abuse is not here. Allow this experi-

ence to be a time capsule where you don't remember the past and the future. You don't need to reviolate yourself by letting them have authority
over you. Don't worry about yesterday. Claim this as your crowning moment. There are rewards." She reports that most embrace this philosophy.

If you are a survivor of childhood sexual abuse or rape, it is important
for you to trust the people around you during childbirth if you are to feel
safe and relaxed. A key to your comfort is having continuity of care from
the same caregivers from the beginning to the end of your labor, and
hopefully from the same caregivers you've been working with throughout
your pregnancy. Given the realities of present-day hospital birth, this almost
certainly requires the services of a doula. It is important for you to establish a basic bond with your caregivers, including a midwife, a doula, and a
doctor, as early as possible in your pregnancy so they can gradually build
your trust. A close relationship between all parties involved throughout all
of labor and birth is essential if a survivor such as you is to have the greatest chance for empowerment and healing during the birth experience.

Although it is always your choice with whom you share information
about your past experience of violation, strongly consider informing
your caregivers so they can be sensitive if any posttraumatic feelings arise
during childbirth. Some survivors find giving birth to their children
healing, as it is both an empowering and sacred experience.

Adding Your Wishes to Your Birth Plan

In this chapter, you've considered interventions and risk management.
You've made a good, wholesome plan that seems appropriate for you
and your situation. If your primary healthcare provider informs you that
you are in a high-risk category, it's especially important to have a full
conversation about the implications for your labor. Ask lots of questions,
and seek a second opinion if you're not satisfied with the answers. If you
are promised that you can have the ideal birth of your dreams, remain
flexible. No one, but no one, can control birth outcomes. Birth is surprising and dynamic.

Set aside some pages in your journal to insert research material on any condition you have that may place you or your baby at risk. Keep copious notes on that topic, and try to learn how many alternatives there are for each of the issues it raises. You'll want to be clear about your preferences in your plan, especially if you're seeking natural birth.

Who is going to stand up for you fiercely, like a warrior, if you need it, and help you get the birth experience you want and deserve? Your birth plan really should include clear instructions for your closest supporters: your spouse or partner, family members, and a doula or birth assistant. Going back to the scientific evidence, do you recall how excellent personal support is one of the main factors in both safety and empowerment during birth? In the next chapter, you'll find out why you need it and how to get it.

T e n

Your Support and Advocacy Team

Doulas, Fathers-to-be, Family Members, and Other Loved Ones

When Laura's son Jesse was born, the situation couldn't have been a more ideal home birth. Her primary midwife lived across the street, and she and Laura were good friends. Although her son was ten days overdue she wasn't put on a steamroller of being induced. Instead, the midwife kept evaluating to see if the baby was being compromised.

When the labor started, Jesse was "posterior," facing her belly instead of her back. For a baby's head to pass through the canal, it's better if such a baby turns. So Laura definitely needed labor support from the midwife and her assistant, as they knew positions that would facilitate the birth. But once labor started, even with this minor complication, it was her husband's support that she remembers most fondly. Laura believes Frank was good at labor support because he worked as a shepherd. He was very patient and kind. "On every contraction, he told me he loved me," says Laura. "The midwives let Frank do most of the physical support, although they stayed in the room and guided him with specific suggestions at the right moments."

When you are considering the number and kind of companions you want to have with you during the birth of your baby, even at a home birth, they may be few or several. During a natural birth at home or in an out-of-hospital birthing center, while midwives are attending to your physical needs, your husband, children, and other family members, for instance, could provide you with tender loving care. So can a doula, a trained birth supporter whose primary motivation is your well-being. Emotional support is highly beneficial to women in labor. Having a loved one (or several) present, focused on the mother-to-be's comfort and concerns above all else during labor not only puts a woman at ease, it also can be truly useful in ensuring that her needs and wishes are met.

The Importance of Support During Labor

Doctors and hospitals are not used to having anyone telling them what they can and can't do, most particularly their patients. It's not that they're uncaring or malicious people, it's just that their attention is set on getting the job done clinically and efficiently. And don't forget, they see hundreds of births every year. You, on the other hand, are going through a significant life passage, an emotional and spiritual event. For this reason, it is essential that you have a support person accompany you to the hospital. This can be your husband or partner, a doula, a relative, or a friend. An out-of-hospital midwife can fulfill this function if you are transferred to a hospital for any reason during a planned home birth or out-of-hospital birth, and if your primary birth attendant is a nurse-midwife based in the hospital, your chances of running into conflicts are greatly reduced, as they adhere to a different model of labor and birth than doctors use.

A major research project sponsored in part by Childbirth Connection concluded that continuous one-on-one support during labor is a remarkable element of maternity care that offers well-established benefits and has no known downsides.[1] Evidence from a number of experimental trials has shown that the continuous presence of an experienced support person not only helps women to avoid or delay invasive interventions, it also reduces or eliminates the need for pain medication, decreases trauma to the perineum, and lessens the probability of forceps or vacuum extraction and cesarean. It is particularly powerful when the woman chooses her own companion and the care begins early in labor. Beneficial care may include the following:

- Helping women with physical comfort

- Providing emotional support

- Offering information

- Helping women communicate their wishes to caregivers

- Interacting with women's partners, as desired by the couple

These results have been confirmed by fourteen independent controlled trials run in several countries and in several settings. *A Guide to Effective Care in Pregnancy and Childbirth* reports: "There was remarkable consistency in the descriptions of the experimental intervention in the various trials: 'Support' included continuous presence, if not for all labor, then at least during the active labor and in 13 trials, specific mention was made that support included comforting touch and words of praise and encouragement. The results of the trials were also remarkably consistent, despite the disparities in obstetrical routines, hospital conditions, the obstetrical risk status of the women, the differences in policies about the presence of significant others, and the differences in the professional qualifications of the persons who provided the support." Furthermore, this one factor increased satisfaction in the birth experience, reduced tension, improved the baby's well-being following birth, and contributed to mother-infant bonding.[2]

Especially in a hospital, where nurses and doctors are not continuously in the room, it can be important for a woman to have an advocate to communicate her wishes to busy staff and to remind staff to ask permission before doing a procedure of any kind. A loved one and/or a doula can put a foot down and raise a ruckus if necessary. They can stand guard at the door and sweet-talk hospital staff. A study reported that a low-risk mother having her first child in a teaching hospital was attended by sixteen people during six hours of labor, but was still left alone most of the time. Another study found that women giving birth in hospital encountered an average of over six unfamiliar professionals during labor, with some women reporting up to fourteen attendants.[3] One home-birth midwife told me that if she transports a woman in labor to the hospital, she always carries a rubber doorstopper with her. She claims it is the most important tool in her possession. Every time someone comes to the door, that person must knock instead of barging right in as usually happens in hospitals. The mother gets to decide who is permitted in and it makes her feel more in charge. Besides being a liaison with staff, the advocate is an emotional comforter—at times, even a "gofer," frequently running errands.

At its physical and emotional best, support for women in labor has always reminded me of dolphin birth. When a dolphin gives birth to a calf, several female dolphins swim in a circle close to the laboring mother. Slightly farther away, another larger group of all the remaining females in the pod also circle around the laboring dolphin. Then, even farther away, all the male dolphins in the pod circle around her. The entire collective comes together to protect the laboring dolphin and her emerging calf from intrusion and harm. A woman giving birth to a baby thrives when she's at the center of a circle of love.

Many women describe sharing the birth experience with their husbands as the ultimate marriage ceremony or a healing experience. In the case of one couple whose baby was in distress during the last moments of birth, the husband stayed by his wife until they knew what had happened. Just beforehand he had told the doula, "No matter what, I need to be there for her!" As the doctors were working on the baby, he said to his wife, "You are more important to me than anything in this world. The doctors are taking care of the baby. I can't help, so I am staying here with you." It was healing for her on the deepest possible level to know she was important and loved, as much so as the baby.

Husbands aren't always able to be as calm as women experienced in birth. As Penny Simkin, founder of Doulas of North America (now DONA International), says, "It's awfully hard sometimes to watch the person you love in pain or frustrated or discouraged with a lack of progress. And there's a tendency to want to rescue her from that. Partners do not have the objective, calm perspective and experience that a woman needs and a doula has."[4]

Taos, New Mexico, is an isolated rural area where the thread of traditional Native American and Hispanic midwives was never lost as the medical model of childbirth gained ground. As a result, it's normal there to have an out-of-hospital, midwife-attended birth. Twenty-five percent of births in the community happen either in an out-of-hospital birth center or at home, and this is culturally accepted as normal.[5] At the Northern New Mexico Women's Health and Birth Center in Taos, birthing women are encouraged to have a doula or at least a calm, loving woman experienced in birth stay with them, in addition to midwives.

It's also a custom in some of the large Hispanic or Pueblo families of Taos for many female relations—the mother, a sister, an aunt or two, a grandmother, some cousins—to be present for a birth. The laboring woman will be working hard, no fooling around, while these women are standing around smiling. Thus, she can tell just by a glance that everything is OK, because of how her family is reacting. If something were wrong, they wouldn't be standing there, would they? A wonderful, nonverbal message is conveyed that the woman is not being traumatized and whatever she's feeling is normal.

Many contemporary women are lucky to have a similar circle of confidence around them.

The Important Role of Doulas

Birth doulas are women experienced in birth who provide continuous support to pregnant women during labor.[6] They receive training to fulfill this special role and have knowledge of the most common birth procedures and the most common problems women encounter. Postpartum doulas provide support during recovery from labor. Doulas do not pretend to be nurses or midwives or doctors, and they embrace the role of giving loving support. A doula can offer nurturance to a woman even when her husband and family are there.

According to the Seattle Midwifery School, which trains doulas, birth doulas assist pregnant women, and, secondarily, their partners, in preparing and carrying out a birth plan. A doula "stays with the laboring mother throughout the entire birth process, providing emotional and physical support and an objective viewpoint. She also helps her clients get the information they need to make informed decisions."[7]

Unless a woman is attended by a doula during her hospital birth, the labor-and-delivery nurses will tend to be the woman's primary caregivers whenever a doctor is not present. In some instances, both a doula and nurses care for the woman—with the doula giving emotional and social support. As we discussed in chapter 3, women do not have a choice of their labor-and-delivery nurses, who rotate according to their shift schedules.

Only 10 percent of hospital births in the United States involve midwives. Given the current situation in hospital maternity wards where overtasked labor-and-delivery nurses don't have the opportunity to provide continuous support, doulas are a godsend. Research clearly shows that the presence of a doula shortens the length of labor and reduces the number of complications.

Some obstetricians don't like having doulas around, at least in part because doulas speak up for the mother. One doula reports, "If I see a doctor coming in holding a plastic package with an amniotic hook I can say to the laboring woman, 'Oh, look, your doctor is here. Doctor, are you doing an exam?' On my client's behalf I ask, 'Does this mean you'll rupture her membranes?' Lots of times the doctor disappears with the hook as fast as he or she got there. Or the birthing woman says, 'Oh yeah, that may be a good idea.' The important point is that she has time to digest the proposition and make a decision about whether or not she wants that procedure done. It's one thing if there's an emergency. It's another if it's just for convenience." A doula is familiar with the mother's written birth plan, so if her obstetrician picks up scissors to do an episiotomy, the doula can remind the doctor that the birth plan specifies no episiotomy.

Doulas must have thick skin, as it is not uncommon for them to be thrown out of the maternity ward. Some unenlightened hospitals actually forbid doulas to enter. Like the labor-and-delivery nurses, doulas have a difficult task: They must walk the fine line between supporting and protecting a laboring woman and adhering to hospital policy.

How Are Doulas Trained?

Training and certification for doulas is generally available through independent midwifery schools. In fact, some midwifery programs require doula training as a prerequisite to becoming a midwife. Topics that are covered in the average curriculum include communication skills, anatomy, birth positions and practices, and hands-on birth support with mentoring. Before certification, doulas typically watch hundreds of birth videos, read many books, and meet numerous women who describe birth experiences of every kind and outcome.

Valuable Questions to Ask a Doula

The organization DONA International suggests the following questions to assess the doula or doulas you're considering hiring.[8]

- What training have you had—and are you certified? (Feel free to go ahead and verify certification status with that organization. Ask the doula to give you the group's contact information.)

- Do you have one or more backup doulas for times when you are not available?

- May I/we meet with your backup doulas?

- Tell me/us about your philosophy on childbirth and supporting women and their partners through labor.

- May we meet to discuss my/our birth plan and the role you will play in supporting me/us through childbirth?

- May we call you with questions or concerns before and after the birth?

Doulas often begin working with women early in pregnancy. As one doula said, "For me the joy is in the journey. Birth is about the mental-emotional challenges and rewards the mother experiences." She describes, "I work with them starting a few months ahead of time. By the seventh month, the belly gets big and they think, 'Oh my god, this has to come out somewhere. It's surreal!' That's why I do nurturing, hands-on prenatal preparation to calm the nervous system and let the mom know she is physically and emotionally supported. Our time together is private time for her to reveal her deepest fears, secrets, and longings. She reveals her expectations of what she wants her birth to be about, what she would like from her partner, what she hopes she can achieve, and what happens if it doesn't happen.

"In helping her to create a flexible birth plan, we talk about her hopes and dreams and where she feels like she may not be able to handle it. The birth journey starts in those early sessions. But by the time she goes into labor we've talked, sometimes weekly, about how well she's going to do. As a result, she feels stronger and more confident, has a clearer sense of purpose, and has high hopes about the experience.

"I teach women to think of their birth plan as a wish list. I can't promise they're going to be 'in charge,' because the baby is. But they will have the power of choice to the degree that the baby allows it. They feel like it's their birth and their wishes and situation."

- When do you try to join women in labor? Do you come to my/our home or meet me/us at the place of birth?

- What is your fee? What does it include? What are your refund policies?

An Underlying Need for Advocacy

Along with giving you comfort, your support person must be ready and able to advocate strongly for your interests, especially when all your energy is consumed by the labor and birth. This individual must be familiar with your birth plan, aware of exactly what it specifies and why. Furthermore, both you and your advocate must know what your rights are in the hospital and the most effective ways to deal with hospital staff.

Hopefully your relationship with your doctor and the hospital will be congenial and cooperative. Yet instances have been known to occur in which disagreements arose that became adversarial. If this were to happen during your labor, understanding your rights would be essential, particularly since too many doctors are unaware of these rights. The legal situation in hospital childbirth is that the hospital is the domain of the doctors, administrators, and whoever owns the hospital. Nonetheless patients have some absolute rights that override the wishes of their doctors and hospitals, including not being given a medication or a treatment against their consent. (You'll find a more detailed discussion of legal issues related to childbirth in chapter 13.)

Many people are under the mistaken impression that when they disagree with their physician about a course of treatment, the doctor has the right to discontinue care. Professional ethical guidelines actually stipulate that a physician may only terminate care after reasonable notice and after providing for necessary interim or emergency care. Physicians who fail to meet these guidelines may be charged with patient abandonment, which is both grounds for a claim of malpractice and constitutes a violation of ethical conduct that could result in the loss of licensure. If ongoing care is required at the time a physician wishes to terminate care—as it is during pregnancy and childbirth—then the doctor must ensure that the patient is transferred to another care provider.

Some legal protections also extend to doctors. You have the right to refuse a recommended treatment, but you do not have the right to demand a treatment that doctors believe is not good medical care, such as an unnecessary surgery, for example.

Having excellent, continuous one-on-one birth support eliminates many of these problems because it slows down the implementation of invasive procedures, medication, and technology. But a doula has no legal standing and cannot offer informed consent on your behalf. In an emergency situation, if you were incapacitated, your spouse or another close family member should be able to sign consent forms for you.

What kind of legal authority—and documentation—do you need to grant your advocates in the case you must be put under anesthesia and cannot express your own wishes? Although actual laws and the formats for such documents vary state by state, it is not difficult to download a healthcare directive off the Internet that would name someone to speak for you. Sometimes these forms are called medical powers of attorney, a healthcare proxy, or a healthcare directive. Or have one drafted by an attorney.

Preparing Your Birth Kit

Once your support team is in place, along with your paperwork authorizing decisions to be made under emergency conditions, I encourage you and your partner to think of the positive aspects of the upcoming experience. Pull together a birth kit of items that will set the mood for a satisfying, inspiring experience at your birth site. Items you might consider bringing include music, pictures, comfortable clothing/pajamas, special snacks and beverages, heating and cooling gel packs, massage oil, a cellular phone, and specialized birth equipment (for example, an Amish birthing stool). After touring the facilities of the intended birth site, you'll know what they've got to offer in the way of equipment and decor.

Adding Your Wishes to Your Birth Plan

Go directly to your birth plan and consider the issue of support. Continuous one-on-one care is the biggest predictor of having a positive laboring experience in any birth location. It's no secret that, as an advocate of evidence-based maternity care, I understand the value of doulas and midwives. But continuous care can come from anyone as long as they are really "with" you, attentive to your physical and emotional needs and concerns, and can make you feel secure and sheltered.

What is your vision for the role of your spouse or partner in the childbirth? And for family and other significant people you know? Being cared for during labor may be symbolic of an entire relationship. How do you dream of being supported and nurtured? Reflect on advocacy in your journal, negotiate with your spouse/partner, and only then inform your caregivers. Use the list of valuable questions to interview doulas, if you want to have one with you in the labor room, and make notes on what's said in your journal.

No birth plan would be complete if it did not include instructions for the immediate care of both you and your newborn baby. Mother-friendly care, in fact, incorporates baby-friendly care. So let's take a look at these issues in the next chapter.

Eleven

Welcome to the World!

Baby-Friendly Hospital Care

"My daughter was born in three or four hours," says Kathy. "It was quick. My water didn't break. I woke up at four A.M. feeling unwell: hungry and as though I was having menstrual cramps. Then I realized that it was the baby. I called the doctor and he said to stay at home as long I could for comfort. Apparently first babies often come slowly. But by six A.M. my husband and I were at the hospital and I was already halfway dilated. I had a vaginal delivery. It hurt a lot, but I was very determined. I pushed as hard as I could for half an hour and she came. Afterward I was exhausted. It is tiring to push so hard.

"I was very happy when I first held my daughter. The nurses took her away for a few minutes so I briefly wondered if something was wrong. But I could see her on a table nearby and she was fine. They cleaned her off, wrapped her up, put a little hat on her, and handed her to me. My husband, who held my hand during most of my labor, was such a proud daddy. In a second I knew it was all worth it. All the kicking, tiredness, sleepless nights, and going to the bathroom every five minutes was worth it. The pain. The bills. Everything. It's the most wonderful feeling to know you created a human being, a life!

The first moments following birth are often exhilarating for a woman, representing the culmination of an incredible physical and emotional journey. These are moments filled with relief from pain and effort, as well as satisfaction and joy. Right then, in a fulcrum where past, present, and future, and all of who you are converge; where celebration or disappointment meets hopes and dreams, exhaustion, and a flood of heightened physical sensations; and when the reality of the tiny, vulnerable stranger lying in your arms is setting in—just when you are ready to rest—hospital staff are very likely to step in and produce a swirl of activity centering on your baby. During this time, it is important to have the support you need from your husband, family, friends, or a doula to help you handle the situation. Events that occur in the first few minutes, hours, and days of a baby's life are critical to that newborn's well-being in infancy and childhood.

What does the scientific evidence show that a newborn baby needs most in order to thrive? To breastfeed and have close contact with the mother. Once your baby is born, your baby's health and yours essentially become a unified entity, so you need to prepare yourself to handle the beginning stage of life by fostering your mother–infant bond. In this chapter, we'll explore how baby-friendly hospitals are organized, as well as routine hospital procedures to look out for that aren't the healthiest ways to care for a baby.

Building the Mother-Infant Bond

One new mother related the first moments after her daughter's birth. "The doctors and nurses at the hospital were very professional, but to me their activities looked like Charlie Chaplin's film *Modern Times*, so I didn't let my daughter leave me. As I was pushing out the afterbirth, my husband stood beside our new daughter across the room from me while they gave her a checkup. They were giving her a vitamin K shot and she was crying, and I saw it from fifteen feet away. So I told the nurses, 'I can walk,' got up, and went over to her. As soon as she heard my voice she stopped crying. Then, my husband and I took her to the room with us. There was a sort of hotel attached to the hospital that has rooms with a double bed for husband and wife, and another bed for the baby.

"We stayed for a day and I got help with breastfeeding from the nurses. My nipples were sore. The colostrum changes to regular breast milk the second day. When that happened, it was as if suddenly, in one minute, I had milk. My breasts got huge and felt like solid blocks. A nurse massaged them, vacuumed some of the fluid out, and put on ice pads. My daughter didn't release from my nipple for nine hours."

According to the safest obstetric and neonatal practices, hospitals should not restrict mother-infant contact when your baby is first born. Your baby should never be taken away from you, not even to do an initial pediatric exam (as was done in both stories above), unless your baby's condition is poor enough to require special care immediately. Even in such cases, initial evaluation should take place in your presence. An examination by a doctor, midwife, or nurse can easily be done with you lying where you gave birth, holding the baby on your chest or with the baby next to you on the bed, so as not to interfere with contact. An added benefit of doing it in your presence is that this provides an opportunity to answer your questions about the baby and also to teach you how to do your own evaluations.

What Exactly Happens During Your Baby's Initial Evaluation?

After your baby is born, a doctor, a midwife, or a nurse who was present at the birth will, of course, want to observe the condition of your new baby. Part of their observation process has been standardized into the "Apgar score," named after Virginia Apgar, M.D., who devised the measurements many years ago. The score, which is charted at one minute, five minutes, and ten minutes after birth, looks at the baby's respiration, heart rate, muscle tone, reflex irritability, and skin color, with a score of ten being a perfect score. In hospitals a nurse usually measures the Apgar, unless a pediatrician has been called in because trouble is anticipated. In an out-of-hospital birth, your midwife takes care of the evaluation.

Your midwife or doctor will also wish to do a medical examination of your new baby within the first hour after birth. This more thorough examination looks for defects, both internal and external, and checks the condition of the heart, lungs, and nervous system. Some hospital delivery rooms are furnished with a special infant examination table and equipment that are kept warm for this purpose. But a much better place to carry out this examination is upon the mother's chest. Research has shown that a baby lying between the mother's breasts has a better heart rate and respiratory rate and a more stable temperature than it does lying on an examination table.[1]

Your participation in your baby's medical exam is essential, as the examiner can demonstrate to you what the exam shows and explain certain characteristics of the baby. As I mentioned above, this affords you the opportunity to ask all the questions you wish with both the baby and the examiner right there, for example, "When my baby was lying on his (her) back, why did you lift the baby up a little ways from the table by its arms and then suddenly let go?" (The examiner will tell you that this is an important test of the baby's neurological functioning.) Your participation is an important introduction to your new baby and, especially if this is your first baby, starts the process of building confidence in your mothering skills.

At birth, a few babies have difficulties and need to be transferred to intensive care. This, of course, means a baby cannot stay with its mother. Unless your baby is in extreme distress, even if your baby needs intensive care, it is usually possible for you to have a few minutes with the baby before it is transferred. When there has been a cesarean section, often your baby can be brought by to see you before the transfer if you are awake. You should request to see your baby if at all possible to take advantage of the opportunity for early bonding.

If your baby's intensive care unit is in the same hospital where the birth took place, you can visit the baby in intensive care. So can other family members. Hospital staff must keep you informed about how your baby is doing. Many intensive care units assign specific personnel just for this purpose. This is important, as involving parents in newborn intensive care is now understood to be an essential component of the care. If your baby is in a different hospital, other family members will need to visit the baby frequently until you are out of hospital and able to come to your baby yourself.

The Importance of Rooming-In

Starting in the mid-twentieth century, hospitals took newborn babies away from their mothers and put them in a central newborn nursery where doctors and nurses could keep an eye on them. Perhaps the biggest pediatric mistake of the last 100 years, not only has this practice created infectious epidemics with significant mortality among babies, it has also interfered with successful breastfeeding and the development of the vital bond between mother and child. Failure to bond has more serious long-term consequences for both mother and baby than almost any other factor in the hospital experience.

There is good evidence of the need for human touch and close contact early in life. An interesting study of low-birth-weight babies in the neonatal ward of one hospital showed that stroking the body and passively moving the limbs for fifteen minutes three times a day for ten days resulted in 47 percent faster weight gain per day, faster maturation, and six days shorter hospital stay.[2] Touch will be good medicine for your newborn, too.

In another study, researchers tested the hypothesis that the amount of crying that people in industrialized societies like ours consider to be "normal" is, in fact, "excessive" and results from not carrying the baby as much during the day as members of so-called primitive societies do. What was the outcome? It turns out that babies who are carried fuss 43 percent less overall and 51 percent less during evening hours. Extra carrying reduces the duration of crying episodes and alters the typical pattern of fussing in the first three months of life. Researchers concluded that the relative lack of carrying in our society might predispose normal, healthy infants to crying and colic.[3]

A baby sling is a valuable piece of equipment because it allows you to carry your baby and still have your hands free. It does not need to be fancy or expensive, just a simple piece of fabric that goes around your neck and cradles the baby either in front or in back of your body will suffice. It is useful to bring one to the hospital so you can take your baby with you wherever you go from day one on.

Today we know that a newborn baby will synchronize its movements with adult speech. Infants that stay in the same room with their mothers regulate the physiological rhythms of their sleeping and waking cycle to their mothers' diurnal rhythms. An infant can distinguish between the voice of a stranger and its mother by the second week of life. But several interactions must happen over a period of days in order for the mother–infant bond to be established and strengthened. It is not immediate.

Formerly, it was commonly held that the bond a woman feels for her newborn baby is purely instinctual. Of course, scores of women felt embarrassed if their personal experience differed from that "ideal." But they weren't abnormal. Bonding takes time. Fortunately, in most cases, central nurseries have been replaced by "rooming-in" all normal, healthy babies with their mothers. Although some hospitals still give a mother the choice between putting her baby in a nursery or rooming-in, since nurseries present a threat of infection and interfere in the creation of mother–infant bonding, giving the family the risky choice of the nursery fails to eliminate this unsafe option.

Benefits of rooming-in include the following:

• Optimal opportunity for contact

• Mom can become familiar with her baby's early signals, needs, and schedules

• Mom can detect symptoms of problems sooner

• Baby cries less

• Frequent breastfeeding, with all the benefits that provides on top of nourishment

• Dad and other family members have a better opportunity to get to know the newborn

• Mom is better prepared to take the baby home as she feels more capable

• Less risk of infection, as baby already has immunity to mom's germs

An Unfortunate Consequence of Central Nurseries

In 1976, an interesting accident happened in Guatemala. An earthquake damaged a large hospital that had a history of persistent infections and newborn deaths in its central nursery. Much of the hospital was destroyed, including the nursery, and so, by necessity, their routine procedure of taking babies away from their mothers was switched to keeping babies in the same bed with their mothers. Space after the earthquake was tight. Even though the beds were crowded together, morbidity due to infections dropped from 17 per 1,000 newborns to 3 per 1,000, and consistently remained at that low level.[4]

Our culture's belief that babies *need* to be placed in a sterile environment derives from the problem of infection that arises when normal, healthy babies are grouped together in hospital nurseries. To counteract the problem that comes from this practice, nurseries have been designed to isolate babies more and more, which heightens the erroneous sense we have that babies *need* to be kept separate. What babies actually need is to be with their mothers.

A mother's body can be as safe, or safer, a place for a tiny baby as an expensive, high-tech machine called an incubator. For more than ten years now, we've had excellent research findings from major university hospitals throughout the world, including the United States, Germany, Sweden, and the United Kingdom, proving that for babies born too small, if they can breathe on their own and are capable of sucking and swallowing—and this includes the majority of premature babies—placing them skin to skin between their mother's breasts and leaving them there twenty-four hours a day, rather than in an incubator, results in fewer babies dying, fewer infections in the babies, better regulation of breathing, more stable temperature in babies, faster growth, and earlier discharge home.[5] This method, called kangaroo care, is widely used around the industrialized and developing world, except in the United States, where many neonatologists have resisted its adoption.

By the way, just as when you're in the delivery room, wearing hospital gowns in newborn nurseries is a Hollywood-style act. Plenty of data prove it's of no value. It only serves to make parents and families feel as if the baby is off-limits. In addition, allowing siblings to visit the newborn in the hospital does not pose a risk to the baby's health. Children generally don't carry dangerous germs, whereas the hospital staff often does. What can truly safeguard your baby's health and boost immunity? Breastfeeding.

The Breastfeeding Decision

Breastfeeding lost popularity in America following World War II due to changes in the culture. Young women lost knowledge of how to breastfeed partly as a result of the increasing isolation between family members. Fewer experienced female relatives lived in the same household to pass on tips to overcome difficulties that arose. Information on infant care originated with doctors and scientists and was based on the medical model in which human beings are granted authority to control and redirect biology.

When we look at women in hunting-gathering societies, we discover that they follow a more natural course. They feed their babies for short intervals thirty to forty times a day.[6] This is appropriate for the design of our species. Because human milk is low in fat and low in protein, babies must feed almost continuously, unlike some animals in the wild whose offspring typically must survive long separation of four to twelve hours between feedings. Of course, forty feedings would be hard to sustain if you were working eight-hour days or longer in a corporate environment. Lifestyle can greatly affect the decision to breastfeed.

Unwittingly, procedures were put into place in hospitals that posed a barrier to natural maternal actions and jeopardized the success of breastfeeding. For instance, the work schedules of hospital staff were allowed to override the needs of mothers and babies to have unrestricted contact. Feedings were arbitrarily scheduled a few hours apart for the convenience of personnel who had to shuttle babies to and from the central nursery.

Every year, an increasing number of scientific studies demonstrate more advantages to *exclusive* breastfeeding for at least the first six months of the baby's life. It has now been proven that even in highly developed countries like the United States—places where you would expect infants above the poverty line to receive adequate nutrition and medical attention—breastfed babies have lower rates of infections and allergies and higher intelligence than bottle-fed babies.[7] In addition, research has proven that certain steps taken in the first hours and days after birth greatly increase the chance for successful breastfeeding. These include laying the baby on the mother's chest right after childbirth and encouraging breastfeeding within the first hour of life.[8]

Problems with Breastfeeding

Some women initially believe they cannot breastfeed, and then learn that they can. There's a wonderful true story that relates to this issue. During a siege of Paris over a century ago, no cow's milk was available. Many women who felt they were not able to breastfeed found that if there was no choice—if their babies were not to starve—they were all able to breastfeed successfully. No women were unable. By the way, the infant mortality rate fell even though they were living under siege conditions. Only a very small number of women truly can't breastfeed for physiological reasons.

Breast milk is the best milk for newborns, even those that are too small or sick. If the baby is too sick to be nourished by mouth, the baby will be fed through an IV or a stomach tube. Otherwise efforts will be made to use the mother's milk. If the mother is able to come to the baby and the baby can tolerate it, the baby may be taken out of the incubator so the mother can nurse it. If the mother is unable to come, she can express (pump out) her milk and it can be brought to the baby for bottle-feeding. If the baby is not able to tolerate breast milk yet, the mother can nonetheless pump her breasts several times a day to keep them making milk until her baby does become able to breastfeed.

It's important to remember a fundamental principle: The breast makes milk to replace what is taken from it. If no milk is taken from it for some days, the amount of milk made slows down and eventually the breasts stop producing milk.

Breastfeeding and Medication

You should be aware that any drug you take may appear in your breast milk. This would include painkillers and antidepressants as well as over-the-counter medications such as for cold relief. Consult your physician before taking medication while breastfeeding.

Baby-Friendly Hospitals

The United Nations Children's Fund (UNICEF) and the WHO have developed a set of protocols for hospitals called the Ten Steps to a Baby-Friendly Hospital based on the scientific findings concerning breast-feeding, and both organizations are promoting these steps around the world.[9] So far, UNICEF has designated more than 18,000 hospitals around the world as "baby friendly." Baby-friendly hospitals are rare in the United States, even though the federal government, women's organizations, consumer advocacy groups, and even a few professional health organizations are promoting them. Forty-eight have been certified as of this writing, and more are added to the roster each year. In order to be designated as "baby friendly," hospitals must prove they are following the ten steps.

What qualities do baby-friendly hospitals have? Baby-friendly hospitals maintain a written breastfeeding policy that is routinely communicated to all healthcare staff, and they train healthcare staff in skills necessary to implement this policy. In the United States, pediatricians, obstetricians, and family practice physicians with privileges at a hospital must be trained for a minimum of three hours in the advantages and management of breastfeeding. Nursing staff with primary responsibilities for helping mothers initiate breastfeeding must have a minimum of eighteen hours of training.

Baby-friendly hospitals also inform all pregnant women about the benefits and management of breastfeeding. They help mothers initiate breastfeeding within one hour of birth. They show new mothers how to breastfeed and how to maintain lactation, even if they are separated from their infants. They practice rooming-in to allow mothers and infants to remain together twenty-four hours a day and encourage unrestricted breastfeeding. To support breastfeeding habits they refrain from giving infants anything to eat or drink other than breast milk, unless medically indicated. Supplemental food and drink is proven to reduce successful breastfeeding. They give no pacifiers or artificial nipples to breastfeeding infants. In addition, they foster the establishment of breastfeeding support groups and refer mothers to them on discharge from the hospital or clinic.

A mother who had a cesarean section after planning for a home birth was very concerned because her baby was taken away from her while she was in recovery from the surgery. "I didn't see my son for an hour, and then it took another hour for me to get to the room, and so it was three hours later when I finally put him on my breast. In the meantime he did need a bottle because his blood sugar fell. When he drank the formula he sucked it down so hard that he sucked the nipple right out of the bottle. Fortunately, I felt like I was able to bond with him. He breastfed well right away. Luckily the process worked for us, but we had to work at it. Even though babies suck instinctively, to make the breasts work with the baby, you have to teach him how to suck on you."

This new mother found the hospital's lactation nurses extremely helpful. They checked on her frequently. She stayed there for four days and the baby slept in a bassinet in the room with her the entire time. When she needed good sleep one time, the nurses removed her son from the room. As soon as she awoke, they brought him back.

Valuable Questions Following Birth

Your birth plan should cover what happens immediately following birth, such as wanting skin-to-skin contact with your baby, rooming-in, no bottle-feeding, and so forth. I would strongly suggest asking questions of the hospital staff prior to your due date and, in fact, during the selection of a birth location. With a healthy baby, there is no need to rush through a series of procedures. If anyone moves to do something differently than what you planned to happen following the birth, like taking the baby into a separate room to do a physical checkup or giving the baby a bottle of formula to drink when you have chosen to breastfeed, try asking some of these questions:

- Would you do the initial examination of my baby in my presence?

- Is my baby permitted to remain in the same room as me at all times?

- Is there any medical reason my baby cannot stay with me?

- If my newborn *must* be taken out of my presence, how will my baby be cared for?

- Exactly who will be providing that care?

- If my newborn *must* be separated from me, when will my baby be returned to me?

- Will I be able to give the baby my breast milk during the separation?

- Are you aware that I have decided on exclusive breastfeeding (bottle-feeding)?

- What kind of help is available for me as I am learning how to breast-feed?

- Exactly who will be helping me?

- How welcome is my family in these experiences?

- Who can visit me and when?

- What might be the physical, mental, and emotional impacts of any invasive drug and/or surgical interventions I have undergone during childbirth (for instance, drug inducement or augmentation, an epidural, vacuum extraction, a cesarean section) on my baby, first as an infant and then, later on, during childhood?

- If I am to be given a medication, will I be told beforehand and informed of any possible effects it may have on breastfeeding and my baby?

Adding Your Wishes to Your Birth Plan

Pull out your journal and set down your thoughts about postnatal baby care. Do you plan to breastfeed or bottle-feed your infant child? What kind of support do you imagine you might need, especially in the early hours and days of new motherhood, when learning how to feed your baby? Depending on how your labor unfolds when the birthday comes, what eventualities must be taken into consideration to suit your preferences? Use the topics in the chapter you've just read and the list of valuable questions as a guideline in your planning process. These are excellent issues to raise in conversation with a midwife, doula, nursing staff in a hospital, and also with your spouse or partner. I also highly recommend speaking with other women about their nursing experiences—what worked, what didn't work, how did they solve dilemmas? Would they agree to be a resource?

Just as birth doesn't end in the delivery room, recovery from birth doesn't end with your discharge from the hospital. Many changes in your body and spirit can take months to heal. It also takes time to reach a new normalcy and establish routines with your baby. What happens and how will you feel in the days, weeks, and months following birth? In chapter 12, we'll talk about the minor hormonal and mood swings that most mothers experience when pregnancy ends, as well as postpartum depression and the grieving process that often occurs when something goes wrong during labor and delivery.

Twelve

Your Recovery Time

*Making the Transition from Pregnant
to Not Pregnant*

"My recollection of the birth experience is hazy," Chris, age forty, told me. "I was drugged. I had a planned C-section because my daughter was breech. It wasn't really my choice. The nurse-midwife who was supposed to attend me in the hospital stepped out and turned my care over to a surgeon. Laboring naturally wasn't presented as a viable alternative. For the pain of surgery, they gave me an epidural and the drug made me sick. I threw up for eight hours. My daughter was taken to the NICU a few minutes after she was born. She was having trouble breathing. Because of the vomiting there was concern my stitches would rip, so I got another medication to control the nausea. They also gave me IV fluids.

"I had the baby on a Wednesday and my husband and I took her home on Sunday. She roomed-in with me after the first twenty-four hours in a bassinet, and the nurses were truly considerate and helpful. People would stop in at intervals to ask, 'How are things going? Do you need help?' They would check my incision and take my blood pressure. They were nonintrusive but available. I had painkillers for a couple of days. Then I felt fine.

"My biggest concern was that my daughter was receiving enough nourishment. It took some practice to learn how to breastfeed properly. My nipples were bleeding. She had two bottles in the NICU the first day, and they fed her intravenously. She seemed so tiny. The second day home a lactation consultant visited and told me how to hold the baby properly. It turned out she had latched on and was sucking in the wrong place. Getting help with nursing is my top recommendation for any woman with a newborn."

When asked what her long-term recovery was like, Chris said, "It was frustrating to have a cesarean when I had prepared for natural birth, yet I never sank into a depression. I had minimal vaginal discharge because of the surgery. My stitches dissolved over the next several weeks. I was told to wait eight weeks before exercising, at which point I started jogging again. I felt fine by six weeks. Because I breastfed I didn't revert to my menstrual cycle for a year—that's normal. Mainly I was exhausted because I went back to work after three months and fed her a lot at night when I came home from the office. After six years, I still have numbness around the line of the incision."

Another mother, thirty-four-year-old Monique, shared, "I felt moody after my son was born. It may have been hormonal, but also I was sad just because I loved being pregnant. For nine months I grew the baby inside me, then the baby was out and I didn't have the tummy anymore. I couldn't rub him. I had heavy discharge for a few days and then, since I didn't breastfeed, I got my first period after a month. During labor I had an episiotomy. That healed in a couple of weeks. My muscles were tired. If I sneezed or coughed, I would sometimes leak pee at first. But I don't care, as I'm so infatuated with him."

Physical changes related to pregnancy don't stop when a baby is born, even though the body begins to restore its natural balance and heal any bruises or wounds that occurred. Among other things, women undergo a series of hormonal shifts. Lactation commences. If you're a mother with older children, you're familiar with what to expect during the recovery period—although each birth is unique. If you're a first-time mother, you don't have visceral knowledge of how quickly or long it takes to revert to *not* being pregnant. Hopefully this chapter can prepare you. And if you are planning a home birth and then end up going to the hospital, it's a good idea to have a broader perspective on recovery.

In this chapter, we'll look at common postpartum scenarios and answer questions you may have, such as: What kind of healing process must occur? How long should it last? What can be done to facilitate healing? What kind of support systems could be needed? No matter what feelings or physical issues have arisen, how can our mother-infant bonding be encouraged in the days and weeks following my baby's birth?

Recovery After Normal, Uncomplicated Childbirth

It can easily be determined that a woman and a newborn baby are fine—unharmed and safe from danger—within three hours of childbirth. That's enough time to monitor the baby's condition and enough of a window to observe any uterine bleeding in the mother. When the placenta detaches from the wall of the uterus, it leaves a raw area. The uterus, which as you know is a powerful muscle, clamps down on its own at this point, naturally assuaging any blood flow. If there were a dangerous hemorrhage, it would soon be evident.

After a planned home birth, the midwife who assists you stays for two to five hours to make sure everything is OK. After that, she makes daily home visits for a week or so. Each postpartum visit will last thirty minutes to an hour. The purpose is to check your condition and answer questions, have a look at the baby together, and perhaps give you an opportunity to grab a quick shower. If your midwife visits, most likely you won't need to hire a postpartum doula, unless you want more help in handling the baby.

You'll be discharged a couple of hours after having a baby in an out-of-hospital birth center if there are no signs of a complication. Remember, high-risk births do not take place in birth centers, so a number of extra precautionary measures truly are not necessary. Furthermore, the midwives that attend labor in these settings understand the value and comfort of being at home surrounded by your family and belongings. A close connection is maintained between the birth center and the home for about a week, and midwives from the center make daily home visits as they would after a home birth.

Hospital births are a different matter. On average, you'll stay in the hospital for twenty-four to forty-eight hours after the birth of your baby, supposedly to rest. During this time, however, you'll be subjected to hospital routines that were designed for supervising the treatment of sick people, even though you aren't sick. In most hospitals this makes it hard to rest. First thing in the morning, your "vitals" will be taken, as that's the protocol. So at 5 A.M., after being up all night with a baby and only just dropping off to sleep, a nurse or intern will come to check your blood pressure, pulse, and respiration. When you are sent home, you'll be entirely on your own, with the exception of the over-the-phone and office-based care of your doctor, which you must initiate. No one from the hospital will contact you. Thus, it is a good idea for a woman planning a hospital birth either to hire a postpartum doula for those early days or to line up a friend, relative, or neighbor to help.

In the first few hours after birth most women want to get some sleep and have a meal. You could be ravenous, as you've put forth great physical effort. During this period it's also important to breastfeed your baby as soon as possible, primarily to give the baby your colostrum, a breast fluid that has special nutritional and immune-building qualities, and to stimulate milk production, as the breast makes only as much milk as is taken out, and secondarily to establish the family unit. Interestingly, this action can symbolically demonstrate to hospital staff that your baby is not their property.

Throughout the first few weeks at home with a newborn, a woman may feel excited, exhausted, and overwhelmed. If you hire a postpartum doula, she will come to the house in the morning after your first night at home. For the first month, she typically makes visits lasting about three hours apiece once or twice a week. Her purpose is to answer questions about baby care and help you to settle into new household routines, as well as taking some of the load off your shoulders while you physically recover by doing simple tasks, such as preparing nutritious meals and possibly doing a little housework. In our modern society composed of nuclear families, where relatives live distant from one another, the postpartum doula takes the place of an extended family.

What Kinds of Aftereffects Are Normal?

Short-term physiological issues you may face after natural birth include:

- *Constipation:* Your bowel movements could be inconsistent for two main reasons. First, the level of fluids in your body has been shifting significantly. Secondly, peristalsis, the rippling motion in the digestive tract that mixes food with digestive juices, is a function of the parasympathetic nervous system, which has been entirely involved in doing something else (having a baby). It can take a few days for the nervous system to revert to its normal operations. Meanwhile, drink a lot of water.

- *Hemorrhoids:* The pressure from carrying your baby and then bearing down hard during labor could cause swollen blood vessels around your anus. These are normal and easily remedied with applications of over-the-counter creams and warm sitz baths. You can manage pain by sitting on a wedge or pillow when lying on your side, or sitting on a rubber or foam ring to support yourself when breastfeeding. Lots of women buy inexpensive children's swimming rings for this purpose.

- *Pain in the perineum:* Sometimes trauma to the perineum is evident. Other times the perineum is intact and trauma is not visible, yet pain exists and persists. It needs time to heal from being stretched and pounded by the baby's head. Local anesthetics in the form of gels, sprays, creams, or foams seem to be the most effective in relieving pain. By the way, women who practiced pelvic floor exercises (Kegels) prior to childbirth are significantly less likely to have postnatal pain in this area after three months.

• *Breast pain:* Especially if a woman chooses not to breastfeed, she may experience significant breast pain from engorgement of the breast with milk. There seems to be little difference in methods of inhibiting lactation between binding the breasts and taking medication. By the third week, binding seems more effective.

• *Sore nipples:* The skin on your nipples is sensitive and may puff up and become chapped from frequently nursing your baby. After a while a woman's body usually becomes inured to any painful sensations of breastfeeding, and most women find it pleasurable. In the meantime, apply cool packs, aim to minimize chafing on the surface of the nipple, and keep the nipples dry by putting a small piece of gauze in your bra and change it frequently. When it is feasible, leave them open to the air.

   By the way, you don't need to be overly concerned about sterilizing your skin where it comes into contact with the baby's mouth. Once you're at home, you'll be in an environment where you and your baby possess immunity. Your skin and nipples are not sterile and do not need to be. Natural secretions from the nipple sufficiently overcome germs. Use basic rules of cleanliness (soap and water) and don't overdo it. Don't scrub, don't use rubbing alcohol (a major irritant), and don't do anything else unless your healthcare provider recommends it for a specific, sensible reason.

• *Hot and cold flashes:* You've had a baby inside of your body for nine months and it's not there anymore. As a result, your body has to suddenly rebalance your hormonal levels. Experiencing hot and cold flashes is normal and nothing to worry about. It usually ends within a few days. Your overall hormonal system will take six months or so to stabilize, and you may anticipate other less dramatic changes.

• *Urinary and fecal incontinence:* Due to bruising and stretching in and around the vagina, you may temporarily be unable to completely control your bladder and bowels. This problem is usually short-lived, unless a woman has undergone an instrumental birth with forceps or vacuum, or has a very large episiotomy incision or tear, in which case damage may be more of an issue.

- *Uterine pain:* With your baby now gone from the womb, it begins shrinking to its regular size. In the process, you may experience twinges of pain that feel more intense during nursing. This makes sense if you recall that some people have success triggering labor by means of sexual stimulation. Nursing produces a similar response.

- *Vaginal discharge:* In the first several days following the birth of your baby, as the rawness from the detachment of the placenta heals, you are likely to have some vaginal discharge, which may range from minor dripping or leakage, to clots the size of golf balls. It's nothing to worry about and should end in a few days. Use sanitary pads to protect your clothing. Whatever you do, do not insert a tampon or anything else into your vagina while it's healing.

- *Reduction of hypertension:* If you had a pregnancy-related condition, such as high blood pressure or preeclampsia, just as soon as the baby emerges from your body that condition will begin to disappear. Once you're not pregnant anymore, the trigger for high blood pressure is gone. With adequate rest, plenty of fluids, and sensible nutrition, you're going to get back to normal pretty swiftly.

- *Stabilization of blood sugar:* So-called gestational diabetes is another condition that should "miraculously" evaporate once you're not pregnant anymore. Your body's glucose tolerance was thrown off by the presence of a baby inside your womb.

- *Postnatal "baby blues":* Emotional instability marked by crying jags, anxiety, and irritability is commonly experienced by women in the first few days of their baby's life. For most women, it fades quickly and should be gone after a couple of weeks. It is also extremely normal to feel anxious coming home from a hospital with the new baby (women fear being isolated, overwhelmed, and the loss of support). For more on postnatal baby blues, see pages 210–212.

Which Painkillers Are Safest for You and Your Baby?

A Guide to Effective Care in Pregnancy and Childbirth offers an evaluation of pain medications.[1] Apparently some analgesic drugs can cause stomach upset. Others can cause constipation. There's also the concern that drugs will be transmitted to the baby through the mother's breast milk. Acetaminophen (for example, Tylenol) is the drug of choice for mild pain because it is largely free of unwanted side effects. Ibuprofen (for example, Motrin, Advil) is anti-inflammatory and very little is excreted in breast milk, so it comes in second. Aspirin is less satisfactory because it can cause bleeding, gastric effects, and goes into breast milk. Codeine, which is used for stronger pain, is relatively unsatisfactory because it quickly leads to constipation.

If you are planning to breastfeed, the same cautions apply to other medications, such as antidepressants and over-the-counter cold remedies, as apply to painkillers. Always consult your physician, midwife, or breastfeeding consultant if you intend to take drugs while breastfeeding.

What You May Need from Your Support Team

Unless you have had a baby before or spent a significant amount of time around other women with newborns, you may feel as though you are fumbling your way through motherhood at the beginning. Aside from your obvious biological ability to reproduce, you probably haven't been trained for this new social role. Especially in the first few days after hospital birth, when professionals are taking care of the baby, a woman can lose confidence in her ability for mothering. Is the baby even her property— or is it the hospital's? Then she goes home and gets cut off from support.

Having someone around you who understands breastfeeding and

how to overcome its problems is extremely valuable in the first weeks and months of your baby's life. With our modern nuclear family, American women no longer have access to supportive, more experienced women. Especially if you are having your first child, it's a good idea to plan to receive this kind of support from your mother, other mothers, older relatives, a postpartum doula, a midwife, or a neighbor. These individuals don't need to be healthcare professionals. Often hospitals and obstetricians put together support groups for new mothers. You can also contact La Leche League (see Resources). Informal networking with people whose company you enjoy can be the most valuable.

Changes can and will occur in your relationship with your spouse or partner. A man cannot nurse the baby. He will probably miss your attention. Many women understandably don't want to have sexual intercourse for weeks after giving birth. You may also feel like your day in the sunshine has ended. As a pregnant woman, you were the center of attention, and now your baby is a featured celebrity. It's good for couples to talk about the changes and how you feel, and to keep on supporting each other. Becoming parents is a huge life transition and it's normal to need a period of adjustment.

Recovery after a Birth with Interventions

Of course there is always a period of healing from childbirth, but new mothers may face physical challenges that are the consequence of treatment they receive during childbirth. Those who've had cesarean sections, for instance, are recovering from major abdominal surgery and will need extra support for several weeks or months. Infections can develop, and so on. If you've undergone any kind of interventions during labor and birth, your recovery may also involve coming to terms with strong feelings about what happened.

Former childbirth educator Leslie Whitcomb states, "I used to do postpartum adjustment counseling with women who had a birth go wrong for one reason or another. Short of the loss of the baby, what really caused them trouble and affected bonding with the baby was their loss of choice. It may have been caused either by their bodies or by the actions of the medical establishment. But the thing for which they needed emotional healing was having the choice of how to give birth taken away from them. Sadly, when the medical establishment runs over a woman she often feels like it's her fault. I noticed that many women didn't get angry with a nurse or doctor who disempowered them, but rather felt like they themselves had failed. To heal, women needed to look at the loss of the childbirth scenario they had planned to experience and grieve.

"There was a need for a woman who had a medically necessary cesarean section, for instance, to look at her sense of failure. Finally, she realized that she was a successful mother because she let herself be cut to have a healthy child. That's the ultimate goal."

What Are the Aftereffects of Taking Inducing and Augmenting Drugs?

As you saw above, in the section on recovery from natural, uncomplicated birth, it's normal to have a little bit of vaginal leakage and spotting with blood after giving birth. Major bleeding, on the other hand, isn't normal and should be cause for great concern. Serious postpartum hemorrhages are slightly more common among women who've had their labors induced or augmented by drugs. This makes sense though, as the purpose of the drugs is to stimulate stronger and faster uterine contractions and sometimes the uterine muscle can run out of gas and lose its ability to contract. The serious hemorrhage usually occurs because the uterus is atonic—meaning it has lost its ability to contract—and therefore isn't shutting down and squeezing against the raw surfaces.

Your healthcare practitioners will give you instructions on reasons you should call them or go to the emergency room in the immediate period following birth. If you do not hemorrhage within twenty-four hours of birth, chances are good that it's not going to happen. It's even unlikely after a few hours. But that's why midwives hang around your home for a while. You're safe to leave the hospital as soon as this threat has passed—in fact, you should leave, as the hospital is full of dangerous germs and sometimes hospital routines may tire you out, and staff can occasionally even do something unwarranted to your body and/or your baby.

Inducing and augmenting drugs are metabolized and out of your system within a few hours of taking them—evidence of this is that your contractions cease. Therefore, they cannot be passed to your baby through your breast milk.

What Are the Aftereffects of Taking an Epidural?

Due to transmission through the placenta, babies whose mothers were given epidural medications tend to be sluggish when they are born. The drugs pass out of their systems within a few hours. However, more than one study suggests that newborn infants born following epidural anesthesia may continue with a mild degree of neurological difficulty for some time after birth.[2] Like the inducing and augmenting drugs, epidural drugs are out of the mother's system within a few hours, so there is no risk of passing them along to the baby again during breast-feeding.

Postpartum symptoms in women having an epidural vary enormously. They range from no aftereffects, to having mild headaches and backaches, to having severe headaches and backaches. About 10 percent of women suffer to one degree or another from headaches and backaches that linger for a few weeks.[3] Occasionally, about 1 percent of the time, the headaches and backaches go on for a year.[4] In rare instances, women have been temporarily or permanently paralyzed from being given an epidural.

What Are the Aftereffects of Instrumental Birth?

During natural birth, a woman becomes bruised and sore. With instrumental birth using forceps or a vacuum extractor, the bruising and soreness she feels are magnified. You can expect pain and discomfort that lasts for weeks, and possibly greater vaginal discharge. Lacerations may lead to longer-lasting urinary and fecal incontinence.

The baby needs time to recover from these invasive, head-squeezing procedures as well. The baby's head is likely to be bruised and swollen after instrumental birth and, for a few days, he or she may be lethargic and less good at nursing than otherwise.

What Are the Aftereffects of Episiotomy?

Natural tears of the perineum produce less pain and bleeding than episiotomies do. Where the doctor or midwife cuts, and then sutures the perineum, there is a wound that has the potential to become infected if you are not careful. Pain may continue for several days. Treat this wound like other surgical wounds: Clean it, don't fuss with it, and keep it dry. Occasionally, the pain persists for months and painful sexual intercourse may result. In this case, see your doctor.

What Are the Aftereffects of Cesarean Section?

Major surgery takes months to heal. Problems that can arise at different stages in the healing process may include bleeding, infections, adhesions (aggressive and binding scarring inside your abdomen), pain and stiffness, and numbness around the surgical site. As with an episiotomy, you should follow the rules of good hygiene in regard to your stitches: Keep the wound clean, dry, and don't fuss with it. If an infection develops, see a medical doctor and do as suggested, which might mean taking antibiotics.

Usually over-the-counter pain medication—acetaminophen (for example, Tylenol) or ibuprofen (for example, Motrin, Advil)—are sufficient to handle discomfort. If you have more severe or persistent pain, speak with your physician. Numbness should go away as your severed nerves heal. You may, however, feel some itching sensations in the process.

Mild exercise such as frequent moving about and walking and stretching of your extremities is important even in the earliest phase of healing, because it reduces the chances of adhesions forming. A common long-term complication of cesarean, adhesions can be avoided if you start moving around and prevent the scars from locking other tissues of your body into place, thus limiting your range of motion. If you feel concerned about what is happening to you emotionally or physically, contact the International Cesarean Awareness Network (ICAN) as they offer mother-to-mother support. (see Resources).

Postpartum Depression

Some women may feel let down or a bit sad after childbirth, and women who had a bad time during childbirth or who have a sick child are even more likely to feel sad. This is natural, and most often it really isn't a medical problem. Postpartum depression has become a kind of catchall term for difficult emotional issues after childbirth. Research studies show that many women have negative feelings about themselves when birth "goes wrong" and when they receive callous treatment from caregivers in hospitals.[5] There is no comparable data for women who have planned home births. Of course, ambivalence and negativity could always be related to factors of motherhood other than the actual birth experience.

Lots of mothers feel mood swings following childbirth, as their hormones are cresting and falling more than usual. Postpartum feelings can range from elation to severe depression and everywhere in between. Around a third of women typically feel sad off and on for several weeks after birth. While many women feel disabling, symptomatic clinical depression months after the fact, only around one or two women per thousand develop a psychosis that requires hospitalization.[6] Clinically, sadness cannot be labeled depression. However, if sadness is severe and persistent, and if a woman's mind is filled with self-destructive thoughts, it's a good idea to see a professional who can assess her condition.

Everyone's hormones respond to trauma, and a woman is going to be more sensitive to both good and bad experiences around the time of birth. Among other things, this can initiate depression in someone who is prone to it. Events can make or break how any woman feels. There may also be social factors to consider. If you feel depressed, please be aware that healthcare providers know you are not pretending to feel bad. You are not a wimp, a sissy, or a failure for hurting. Your feelings are probably triggered by hormonal shifts and can be regulated through diet, exercise, rest, and support. Medication would be a final solution and does not generally need to be prescribed for life transitions. (See chapter 11 for a discussion of medication and breastfeeding.)

What can you do to cope with strong feelings? Data from different kinds of studies show that the presence of a doula in labor and in the early period following birth significantly decreases the risk of postpartum depression.[7] Cesarean section is a risk factor for depression,[8] as are having a difficult birth and lack of family support. Isolation of a new mother, someone who is hormonally destabilized, exhausted, and overwhelmed by her circumstances, is a strong risk factor. Therefore, seek company. Find someone genuinely supportive to listen to your feelings without judgment. This can make a big difference. Join a group of other women like you who have infants and want mutual support. Your doctor, midwife, hospital, or birthing center may be able to help you locate such a group. Or you could search for a group of like-minded women on the Internet (see Resources).

When Something Goes Wrong

With the modern advancements in care, most parents are not prepared for the experience of a pregnancy or childbirth that goes wrong. Nonetheless, things can and do go wrong. Women and babies are hurt and occasionally die. At such times, parents grieve and it challenges their faith in God, doctors, medicine, technology, and in their ability to produce a normal child. Acute grief is normal and includes restlessness, anger, pining, and anxiety. Someone engaged in grieving may have low energy, bad moods, social withdrawal, impaired memory and concentration, disturbances in appetite and sleeping, and feel a lack of purpose. A strong social network and emotional support is essential to overcoming bereavement successfully in due course.

When a baby is impaired or ill, bonding is made more difficult. It's sometimes hard for parents to accept a child that's not healthy right away or has a disability, and parents may have anxiety about how to handle the situation. The neonatal unit in the hospital is not home, and parents may feel disoriented visiting their baby there. However, the doctors and nurses who work in neonatal units encourage mothers and fathers to come into the intensive care nursery where they may hold and feed their baby.

Some evidence suggests that fathers may recover from grief faster than mothers. There may be difficulties in a marriage at that moment when emotional states diverge. Certainly, many couples are able to pull together beautifully in the face of adversity. No shame exists in asking for counseling or other forms of support. When a baby is sick, injured, or disabled, parents must take good care of themselves so they can be useful to the child. There are many different support groups on the Internet for the parents of children with the same types of disabilities. Other parents can prove to be a great resource of emotional support and practical information.

Adding Your Wishes to Your Birth Plan

With the topic of recovery, we have nearly reached the end of our journey together. Your birth planning process needs to encompass this postnatal period as well as the actual birth experience, because the two are conjoined matters. Not only is it impossible to predict when and how a baby will be born—even elective surgery may surprise you and poses risks of complications—you also cannot predict exactly how your recovery will unfold. But if you hold all potentials in mind, and understand the consequences of earlier choices that linger long past the few hours of labor and childbirth, your plan should feel more complete.

In the next chapter, I'll encourage you to get specific about your wishes, and pin them down on a piece of paper. We'll go over general guidelines for writing a birth plan (some are long and others brief), sample language on specific topics, and legal matters. Before reading on, take this opportunity to write down your feelings about the recovery phase in your journal. What kind of support network would you like to put into place beforehand?

Thirteen

Ensuring Your Wishes Are Honored

Your Plan in Action

A midwife phoned the hospital because a woman under her care for a planned home birth was having a breech (feetfirst) baby. After discussion, it was agreed that the woman should be transported to the hospital. The midwife came with the woman and stayed for the entire birth. The woman arrived with a two-page birth plan, worked out with her midwife, filled with things she wanted *not* to be done, including a C-section—except as a last resort. The obstetrician on call came to see the woman and flat out told her she *must* have a cesarean section. The result was that the woman refused to be under the obstetrician's care. The hospital respected her wishes and another obstetrician was called.

The second obstetrician asked the woman if she would agree to an ultrasound, carefully explaining how it would help everyone to see the exact situation the baby was in. The woman agreed and she and the doctor observed the breech position together. The doctor explained why she thought a cesarean would probably be necessary, but made it clear that it was the woman's choice. The woman said she would think it over and agreed to have continuous electronic fetal monitoring in the meantime. After four hours of her "thinking it over" the monitor began to show signs of fetal distress. The woman was told. Then she agreed that cesarean was a good idea and it was done. Mother and baby were fine, the technology was used appropriately, and the woman's choices were honored.

Though the woman didn't get the exact outcome she hoped for, her planning was intrinsic to her understanding of her baby's birth as a successful, positive event.

Sheryl Rivett, author of *Mothers and Midwives*, served on an official advisory board discussing maternity-care regulations for the state of Virginia. At first the senior policy analysts who were her colleagues couldn't understand who hires and supervises the midwives. She and the other home-birth advocates told them, "Pregnant women are in charge." "But who can we call to check the midwives' references?" some of the board members persisted. "The women." Midwifery was as unfamiliar a paradigm in that room as it is for many among us who weren't taught that mothers are responsible for childbirth.

If you are pregnant, you probably feel a natural urge to protect your baby. Maybe you've stopped smoking or cut down on drinking alcoholic beverages, or switched to organic foods to avoid chemicals; maybe you've stopped cleaning out your cat's litter box to prevent exposure to bacteria; and maybe you've joined a yoga class to stretch and strengthen your body in preparation for labor. Pregnant women undergo real physical and emotional transformations. Beyond imagining themselves in the role of a mother, they dramatically alter their eating, sleeping, exercising, and other patterns. Their commanding internal drive is toward health and security. Taking good care of a baby begins long before labor starts, and it continues for years afterward. Although both moms and dads feel protective, childbirth is a mother's defining act. So, at this point, the man in your life, your family, and your caregivers must follow your leadership.

Throughout this book, you've been weighing the advantages and disadvantages of different decisions involved in childbirth. After reading the information, sit down with your spouse, significant other, or another trusted person to discuss what you have learned, and how it influences your wishes and concerns. (Of course, you may feel comfortable making decisions on your own.) Maybe you feel inspired to change your birth location or primary caregiver. Perhaps some red flags have gone up over certain issues. Hopefully, your priorities are now clearer, and you feel emboldened to ask for what you truly desire. The birth of your baby can be an intimate, sensual event that is a special gift to everyone on hand.

By now, I hope you understand that a birth plan is an approach to childbirth, one that puts the woman in labor at the center of the experience, rather than a term for a specific kind of outcome. Currently an overwhelming majority of American women give birth in hospitals, yet obstetricians and hospitals have important lessons to learn from midwives. As Ina May Gaskin says, "Having a midwife *is* a birth plan." While I generally concur with that viewpoint, in this chapter I will nonetheless explain why adding the birth plan to your medical chart and files can serve as leverage to ensure that your plan is followed, especially if you are planning to give birth in one of the occasional less-than-mother-friendly and -baby-friendly environments we've talked about. In addition, the plan gives you legal recourse against malpractice. Your wishes should be paramount.

Although hostile hospitals and healthcare personnel are the exception, not the rule, I hope you will have the courage to fight for your birth plan if you must.

An Invitation to Greet a New Life

Most women and their partners perceive a birth plan as an invitation to share a beautiful, heart-opening experience with them: welcoming a new life into the world. Families understand the positive sentiment and conviction behind plans. But, strangely, for some professionals, birth plans are controversial documents. Some doctors and hospitals dislike birth plans because they have well-established routines in place for the daily running of the maternity ward and prefer women who comply with these routines, forgetting that this is not another sick patient and that childbirth is not a medical procedure. They find the whole notion of a plan adversarial or they don't want a layperson—not even the pregnant woman whose impending labor the plan describes—to tell them how to get the job done, demonstrating a lack of respect.

Some midwives also dislike birth plans—not so much because they fear lawsuits or participating in woman-centered childbirth—but because they believe birth plans set up rigid and unreasonable expectations for their clients about the course of labor and birth. Clients might be disappointed if things don't go exactly as they imagined.

You may ultimately decide that your birth plan is best suited for your educational purposes or only as an adjunct to certain conversations with your caregivers, rather than as a legal document you want to have signed by your doctor or midwife and added to a medical chart. That is your call. You may also choose to write the birth plan in nonadversarial language (so as not to create unintended and counterproductive friction) and draw upon the plan when applying negotiation skills. Ideally, there is a middle ground. Maybe women and caregivers can simply decide *respectfully* to be on the same team.

If you have reached this point in the book and recognize that your caregiver is so authoritarian that he or she would be unwilling to review, much less sign or honor, a birth plan, my hope is that you'll seriously consider replacing that practitioner with someone more reasonable—or more like-minded. You are the consumer, after all. You pay the bills.

Still, the process of writing a birth plan is about more than outvoting stubborn caregivers. Having a birth plan can help compassionate caregivers to provide you with continuity of care in an environment, such as a hospital, in which many staff members deal with one laboring woman in shifts. If your plan is attached to your chart, they can see exactly how best to help you when any decision needs to be made. They can check in with you and support you with options that make sense according to your plan—and, as professionals, they have the experience and information to do so appropriately. Many hospital staffs welcome a birth plan, as a plan makes it easier for them to provide you with optimal care.

Sometimes women are stuck with primary caregivers who are terrible listeners and rigid adherents to the conventional mind-set—stuck perhaps because they live in a remote, rural community with few practitioners from among whom to choose or because of limitations in their insurance policy or HMO, or maybe due to another reason. If you're one of these women, you need to know that not all doctors and nurses are lovey-dovey about birth plans. The idea is to negotiate your wishes in a way likely to succeed. If you believe you could attract a doctor's wrath and indifferent or bad care by submitting a written plan, by all means keep your birth plan a secret and express your wishes verbally.

Regrettably, when you have few choices of birth attendants in a community you may end up forced to compromise on certain matters. It's important to know both your negotiables and your nonnegotiables, and the planning process can help you make that assessment. Use the birth plan to square away your priorities in your own mind.

The good news is always that most births turn out just fine. When you are working with an excellent, woman-loving obstetrician or an excellent, woman-loving midwife, defensiveness, control struggles, animosity, and improper behavior just don't enter the picture. Most caregivers want women to feel relaxed, supported, and fulfilled during childbirth. It is hard to be present at a birth without being awed by the life force.

Reviewing Your Journal And Options

Way back, at the end of chapter 1, you began recording your thoughts, feelings, and impressions about the topics we've explored together in an informal journal. This would be a good time perhaps to pull that journal out and reread it. Even if you have not kept a journal, you may also benefit from going back to each of the preceding chapters and reviewing their contents. As you do, allow yourself to imagine yourself actually having the childbirth experience and what it's like. Let the consequences of your various options play out in your mind's eye.

- If you knew that everything would go smoothly and safely from start to finish of the labor and birth, what would your ideal scene be? Give yourself the best of the best in this visualization. Would you labor using a birth stool? Would your baby be born underwater in a bathtub? What are your personal preferences?

- If you knew that something would go wrong or would pose a difficult challenge during a portion of the labor and birth, what would your ideal strategy and scenario for handling that problem be? How would you want your midwife or doctor to speak with you? How would you like your spouse or another support person to help? What alternatives would you like to try, and in what order? Again, in your mind's eye, permit yourself to have the best. What would help you relax and be able to continue labor under difficult conditions?

General Guidelines for Writing Your Birth Plan

Remember, your birth plan is a wish list. Its purpose is not to control birth itself, since birth, as a force of nature, is actually under no one's control. Rather the birth plan aims to educate you, help you make decisions and communicate them to your caregivers, and thus, to influence the care you receive. With any luck, your birth plan will help you gain some measure of control over how you are treated during your birthing experience. When women in labor are relaxed and trust those around them, birth outcomes improve.

Add a line at the bottom of your birth plan for your doctor or midwife, and other caregivers, to sign your plan under the statement "I have read this plan and understand it." When caregivers sign your birth plan, they are only acknowledging to you—on the record—that they have read and understood it. They do not have to sign and say: "I agree." No matter what you tell them, they are always responsible for offering you their best judgment and skills as different circumstances arise, and then together you and your caregivers can agree on your care. This benefits you. Your birth plan will help you take responsibility for your decisions and ask to be fully informed.

Here are a few tips to keep in mind as you create your birth plan.

A well-constructed birth plan should be flexible. Birth is a cooperative process and many possibilities could arise. Be flexible. Don't set yourself up to think of your birth as a failure or set up your caregiver as your enemy by rigidly adhering to one—and only one—concept of how it can turn out. Include phrases that show you understand that what is appropriate in one circumstance may not be in another, such as the following:

— "As long as there are no definite signs that I or my baby are in trouble . . ."
— "If circumstances allow . . ."
— "Unless there is an emergency . . ."

Be brief. Keeping the length of your final version of the plan down to one page, or two pages maximum, increases the likelihood that there will be time for everyone on staff at the hospital or birth center to read it and also to be able to remember your specific requests. Of course, the working draft of your plan may be much longer than the final copy you attach to a hospital or birth center chart—and more emotional, personalized, and descriptive. Writing a longer detailed version for yourself, your spouse or partner, and your doula, or another advocate present to support you, is a wonderful idea. Your support team knows you intimately and can be enlisted to get fierce on your behalf if ever the need arises.

One woman laboring in a hospital had clearly told the staff she didn't want a routine IV; nonetheless, they were determined to place a line in her hand. She had her six-foot-two husband assert her point of view by getting in the way of that business. Told that it was "hospital policy," she responded, "I'll rip the line out. I prefer to drink fluids." She figured correctly they wouldn't go to the trouble of having five people hold her down and forcibly insert an IV against her expressed wishes.

Whenever possible state your plan in the positive rather than the negative. The plan should not only be a list of what you do not want done. Positive phrasing reduces resistance on the part of caregivers to honor your requests. For instance, on the topic of episiotomy you could write, "I wish to keep my perineum intact; however, if it comes down to a choice, I would prefer to tear rather than to have a surgical cut."

Phrase your wishes as requests, rather than commands. "We (or I) would like to be given the option of . . ." "We (or I) request that . . ." It is not a good idea to write an adversarial or dictatorial birth plan, because professionals may find them threatening. Being put on the defensive reduces their ability to listen and respond.

Be as specific as possible. Suggest your preferred alternative from the research you have done. For instance, on the subject of anesthesia during a cesarean section, you could write: "If a cesarean section becomes necessary, we (or I) request, if circumstances allow, that I be given an epidural rather than a general anesthetic."

Making Note of Your Basic Preferences

Prior to drafting the words of your plan, use the following lists of subjects to define your preferences during every stage of labor, birth, and following birth, and guide conversations with your caregivers. I've included a few examples under each topic to illustrate what you might decide to write, but feel free to develop your own language. These are merely samples.

On the Subject of Informed Consent

Legally, before any medical procedure may be done, you are entitled to fully informed consent, meaning you must be given the full facts on risks and benefits. Although a signed birth plan has no legal influence unless something goes wrong during childbirth, as a social document a birth plan has great value to you, because it puts the onus on your care providers to follow your plan in case problems arise. A birth plan brought to a hospital or birth center by a pregnant woman has the legal status of a consent document, meaning that it describes to what she will and won't consent. Thus, if something isn't specifically featured in the birth plan, the legal assumption is that the woman has not consented to the procedure. For this reason, it is important that you sign your plan.

Under the law, your authority over your body is absolute except if you're unconscious or incoherent. When you're not able, a spouse or other family member is granted this authority by law—check your own state's law to be sure—whereas a nonrelative would need a valid, written legal directive. Who do you choose to speak for you if you are incapacitated and an important decision must be made? Put it in your plan.

Consent. Include the following types of phrases in your birth plan and in your verbal communication with care providers.

—"Fully informed consent . . ."
—"What are the known risks of . . ."
—"We need time to make this decision . . ."
—"Are there any alternatives?"
—"Thanks for explaining that option; we will consider that."
—"We need more information."

Medical directives. Add this type of language to your birth plan: "In case a decision about a medical procedure, such as a hysterectomy following a cesarean, may be made when I am unconscious, I grant the authority for making that decision to my husband (or other individual)."

Healthcare proxy. A healthcare proxy is a document that designates someone to make healthcare decisions on your behalf if you become incapacitated. You should *always* have a medical proxy with you, a signed document that may (or may not) need to be notarized depending on the state in which you reside. Proxy laws vary from state to state; they are not national in scope. It's critical that your healthcare proxy is immediately available in case an urgent situation arises. Consider adding this to your medical file along with your birth plan before or as you check into the hospital or birth center.

On the Subject of Location and the Labor Environment

Where will you give birth, and how do you want that environment to be? Some pregnant women and their partners prepare one plan for their planned home birth, and another plan in case it becomes necessary during labor to transport the woman to the hospital.

Location. At the top of your plan you might indicate that you are planning a home, out-of-hospital birth center, or hospital birth, and add the name of the institution:

—"I am planning a home birth. Below follows a description of how I would like my birth to happen, and what I would like in case of various emergency contingencies. . . . I understand that there may be circumstances in which it is necessary that I be transported to a hospital. Some of these situations are un-ambiguous (for example, hemorrhage, severe fetal distress) while others are judgment calls. While it needs to be a joint decision, I will rely heavily on my attendants' expertise in these matters. My primary concern is that the baby and I come out of the process as healthy and happy as possible."

—"Birthplace: Home."

—"Birthplace: Birth Center."

—"Birthplace: Hospital."

—"Birth site: Family Birth Center at Reliable Hospital in (spec-ified town, state). My goal is to deliver my baby as safely and naturally as possible without medical interventions unless the benefits outweigh the risks."

—"If everything is processing well and normally, I am planning an underwater birth at the Independent Birth Center with the assistance of a midwife."

—"To the staff at Memorial Hospital: My husband and I under-stand that childbirth is full of surprises and that decisions may need to be made in the labor room. We intend to work with everyone present to make good decisions if need arises. The following items are our preferences if the birth goes smoothly."

—"We realize that some of our choices in childbirth aren't common in some hospital settings, and we thank the obstetri-cal staff for respecting our wishes."

Labor room. Explain your preferred environment in a sentence or two:

—"We'd like to have the same room for labor, birth, and imme-diate postpartum if possible."

—"No bright lights or loud noises, please."

—"Lighting: dim."

—"I have chosen to labor with soft music playing to promote meditation."

—"The ground floor of our home will be open to family and friends as childbirth takes place upstairs; however, we ask that everyone other than the labor support team stays in the kitchen/living room area and keeps the volume down."

On the Subject of Birth Attendants and Companions

Who will help you, and how would you like them to behave?

Primary caregiver. Simply add a line labeled "Birth attendant(s)" or "Primary care provider(s)" and insert the names of the doctor or midwife you've chosen. If you wish, you may also list the backup caregivers.

—"Birth attendants: Mona Simpson, CNM, and Marge Simp-son, CNM."

—"Family practitioner: Dr. Melissa Simpson."

—"Obstetrician: George Nathaniel, M.D."

Companions/labor support. This category might include your husband, mother, father, sister, friends, older children, and so on. It's a good idea to specify these people by name and indicate your relationship to them:

—"Labor support: Mack Macintosh, husband and father-to-be. He is to stay at my side at all times, even in an emergency."

—"I prefer for my husband and mother to be present at all times. All other companions, such as friends, will be decided on the spur of the moment."

—"We reserve the right to kick anyone out of the room at any time."

—"No interns/apprentices, or others in training, should enter the birth room without explicit permission."

Doula. A doula might be listed as labor support or have her own line in the plan:

—"I'd like my doula, Mary Macintosh, to stay by my side at all times, even in an emergency."

On the Subject of Basic Care

How do you want to handle the basics of your care? Various elements in this category may overlap with one another.

IVs.

—"No routine IVs."

—"IV only in the case of dehydration or for the administration of medication."

Food and beverages.

—"I am planning to eat light snacks and drink clear fluids throughout labor."

—"Nourishment: Soup and sandwiches. Beverages: clear fluids and ice chips."

—"To balance my electrolytes and keep up my strength, I'll drink a combination of sports drinks, smoothies, broth, and water."

Electronic fetal monitors.

—"Intermittent fetal monitoring except in case of severe fetal distress."

—"I would like to wear a portable monitor that does not interfere with movement."

—"Monitoring: Use of a stethoscope or Doppler."

Clothing. Do you prefer to wear clothing of your own, hospital garments, or be naked? Include it in your plan. With home birth this isn't an issue; however, you might wish to pack your bag with a few clothing options.

Vaginal examinations.

—"The minimal number required for you to assess my progress."

—"Staff should please ask my permission before doing a vaginal exam, and explain why it is necessary. I would also like to know what you found out afterward."

Special religious or cultural requirements. Is there something sacred or ceremonial that you need to do or say, or in which you would like to involve your birth attendants? Include it in the plan.

Special needs. Some women have physical or emotional conditions about which caregivers need to be made aware. For instance, if you are legally blind and have concerns about your vision and eyeglasses, those should be included in your plan—or perhaps you are deaf or wear a prosthetic limb and wish to have extra assistance at a given stage of labor. If you are an abuse survivor and need to be handled very gently, put that need in your birth plan with an explanation of how to handle it.

Videotaping/photography. Some maternity-care facilities discourage videotaping, in which case you need to let them know ahead of time that this is part of your plan.

Making Note of Your Preferences for First-Stage Labor

As you are aware, early labor can last for days or hours. First-stage labor is the period of time in which your cervix is dilating. Once regular contractions begin, it's a good idea to notify your primary caregiver and decide when you will go to the hospital or birth center, or when your midwife will come to your house. Different issues can be involved.

On the Subject of the Onset of Labor

Natural labor can begin in a number of ways, such as by the amniotic sac breaking, or by the gradual onset of contractions. If you are over two weeks "postterm," your primary caregiver will be on the alert for placental malfunctions. If your water breaks, your caregiver will watch you for signs of infection. Here are some issues that you may choose to include in your birth plan.

Induction of labor.

—"No induction of labor."
—"Spontaneous onset. If it is delayed or there are complications, we would like to discuss our options at the time."
—"Under no circumstances whatsoever should I be given Cytotec." (This statement applies to both cervical ripening and induction.)

Membranes/water breaking.

—"No artificial rupturing of membranes without first explaining why and getting my permission."
—"If my water breaks, I plan to remain at home for at least twenty-four hours, resting quietly, until I have regular contractions or develop a fever."

Antibiotics.

— "Unless there are definite signs of infection, I'd prefer not to receive antibiotics."
— "If my water breaks and I am not fully dilated for a long stretch of time, I'd like to discuss the pros and cons of taking antibiotics."

On the Subject of the Progress of Labor

Watching the clock—the arbitrary assignment of time frames for any stage of labor—is proven to lead to an increase in unnecessary interventions. You may wish to add language to your plan in order to avoid this increased risk.

Speed of dilation.

— "I prefer to try natural methods to promote dilation, such as walking and sexual stimulation, rather than taking drugs."
— "We do not wish labor to be hurried, unless signs show our baby is in trouble."
— "My midwife and I have discussed cervix-softening herbal remedies, and I may choose to take them if dilation seems to be prolonged."

Augmentation with Pitocin or other drugs.

— "Except for an emergency, I do not wish for my labor to be augmented."
— "If there is an apparent need to speed labor, please explain all my drug and nondrug options to me at the time."
— "If my caregivers and I agree that augmentation is necessary, I would only agree to Pitocin for this purpose."

On the Subject of Pain Management

Labor pain is one of the more tricky issues in childbirth, because it stirs up fear in many women and yet scientific evidence shows it plays a valuable role in the progress of labor. There are many different ways of handling it, and you need to form a clear strategy.

Natural pain management.

— "Pain management: I plan to use a combination of self-hypnosis, deep breathing, and acupressure to manage my labor pain."
— "I am having a natural birth. Please do not offer me any pain-relieving medications unless I specifically request them."
— "To relieve pain, my partner and doula will help apply counterpressure and hot and cold applications of gel packs."
— "My preference for pain relief is to immerse myself in water."
— "With the guidance of my doula, I intend to handle the pain of my contractions using an active visualization process."

Epidural.

— "Before pain medication is given, I would like to meet with the anesthesiologist to discuss all my possible options for epidurals and analgesics."
— "Epidural should only be offered to me if I am taking an augmenting drug."
— "I would like to have an epidural under the following circumstances . . ."
— "If I appear to be suffering and exhausted, and labor seems emotionally traumatic, then let's discuss the risks and benefits of a short-term epidural."
— "As an abuse survivor, I would prefer to receive strong pain medication to avoid my contractions stirring up renewed feelings of trauma."

On the Subject of Movement

Your planned activities might include walking and dancing, as well as bouncing on a birth ball or shifting spontaneously. Movement can provide relief from discomfort.

—"Freedom of movement is important to me, as I am planning to move freely during the first stage of labor."

—"During the birth of my last child, I was most comfortable bouncing on a birth ball. My plan is to sustain rhythmic activity of this sort again to help my pelvis open wide and assist my baby's passage through the birth canal.

—"Unless there is a serious contraindication, I don't wish to be still or lie in bed."

—"In stage one, I plan to walk the corridors of the hospital."

—"I plan to let my body guide me to the most comfortable positions during labor and birth, and so I need to be unfettered by technology."

On the Subject of Laboring Positions

Scientifically, the on-the-back, or lithotomy, position has been shown to be the least helpful of any position for the laboring woman.

—"Labor positions: I am free to try whatever works."

—"If I must labor in bed due to being monitored or having an IV line attached to my arm, I would prefer to labor on my side."

—"No lithotomy, except in the case of an instrumental procedure."

—"Gravity-enhanced and vertical positions."

—"I plan to labor by squatting, sitting on a beanbag, or on my hands and knees."

—"With my first birth, laboring on the toilet was most comfortable for me, so I plan to try the sitting position again."

Making Note of Your Preferences for Second-Stage Labor

The second stage of labor lasts from the time you are fully dilated until the baby emerges from your body.

Speed of Delivery. As we discussed in chapter 1, there are good reasons to adopt an attitude of patience during second-stage labor.

—"No watching the clock. I prefer for my baby to be born in his/her own time."

—"Please allow my perineum time to expand around my baby's head as it is crowning. As long as there are no signs of fetal distress, I would prefer not to rush the baby out."

—"As long as the baby is OK, I am not overly fatigued, there is no pain at my earlier cesarean site, and my contractions are continuing productively, I ask that my second stage of labor be allowed to continue without intervention for as long as it takes, even if it is four hours or more."

On the Subject of Instrumental Birth

Here is a checklist of possible considerations:

Consent.

—"If it seems that the baby is stuck in the birth canal, I would like to be fully informed of all my options, including alternatives to using forceps or a vacuum extractor. Please be prepared to explain to me why you would prefer to use an instrument at this juncture, as opposed to doing something else."

Forceps and vacuum extraction.

—"Vacuum extraction is preferred to forceps."

—"No instrumental birth, except as a final recourse."

On the Subject of Tearing and Episiotomy

Here is a checklist of possible considerations:

Consent.

—"I would like to keep my perineum intact. If my care provider believes there is indication for an episiotomy, I want to fully discuss benefits, risks, and possible alternatives before I agree to it."

Massage.

—"I request that the doctor, nurse, midwife, or assistant massage my perineum before and especially during the pushing stage to reduce the possibility of tearing." (Some caregivers use vitamin E oil for this purpose.)

Hot compresses.

—"I request that the doctor, nurse, midwife, or assistant apply hot compresses to my perineum before and especially during the pushing stage to reduce the possibility of tearing." (This could be combined with massage suggestion above.)

Fetal distress.

—"I would prefer not to have an episiotomy unless forceps must be used."

Pushing.

—"My body knows instinctively how to push. I would prefer to push without any comment from my birth attendants or support team. Do not tell me to push or not to push."
—"My husband is working with me during labor and I'll be focusing on his voice as I push."
—"While I am bearing down, please encourage me with supportive statements like 'You're doing great,' 'You can do it,' and 'Hang in there.'"

On the Subject of Cesarean Section

Here is a checklist of possible considerations:

Consent. Even if a cesarean is recommended, there's usually time for consideration.

—"If a cesarean needs to be done, it may not be done until I agree to it. We (I) want to discuss any problems and the associated risks unless there is an immediate medical emergency."

Second opinion. You may locate a professional of your choosing ahead of time, especially for a high-risk birth.

—"It is my strong wish that I give birth vaginally. If my primary care provider determines that a cesarean delivery is indicated, I would like to obtain a second opinion from another physician of my choosing if time allows."

Anesthesia. Three forms of anesthetic are common in the case of cesarean section. Often a sedative is given to calm the mother beforehand. Then, either an epidural is given so the mother can remain awake during the surgery or a general anesthetic is given that renders her unconscious. (Review chapter 7.)

—"If a cesarean section becomes necessary, I would like to have a conversation with the anesthesiologist before surgery to discuss my options."
—"I would prefer to be awake during the procedure if it is medically reasonable."
—"I would prefer to be sedated (or not sedated) before a cesarean."

Partner's presence. Let caregivers know whom you would like in the room during the surgery, including your spouse or partner, midwife, and/or doula.

—"In the event a cesarean section is necessary, my husband will accompany me."

—"I would like my doula, Mary Smith, to stay by my side in the event of surgery."

Participation. During cesarean, there is usually a screen erected to hide the procedure from your sight. Would you like to have your caregivers lower the screen or hold up a mirror at the moment of the actual birth?

—"I would like to view the birth of my baby under any conditions."

—"Though I would prefer not to be able to see the majority of the surgery, I would like the screen to be lowered so I may observe the actual moment of birth."

Contact with the baby. Would you like your baby to be handed to the father or someone else as soon as it is born? Would you like to be shown the baby immediately?

—"Following a cesarean, if the baby's condition permits, we would like the baby to be given directly to my husband. He will stay with the baby while I go to recovery."

Making Note of Your Preferences for Third-Stage Labor

You're in third-stage labor from the moment your baby is born until the placental tissues are expelled from your birth canal. Right away there are some decisions to make about the care of your baby and your own recovery.

Cutting the umbilical cord.

—"We choose to wait to cut the umbilical cord until after it stops pulsing."

—"If he wants, my husband will have the option to cut the cord."

—"Our plan is to harvest some blood and stem cells from the umbilical cord in case of future need."

On the Subject of Baby Care

Here are a few issues for consideration.

First baby exam. Many parents' plans include explicit instructions for treatment of the baby during the initial examination. So consider how you feel about suctioning the baby's nose and mouth, vitamin K injections, antibiotic ointment for the eyes, and so forth.

—"Initial evaluation of our baby should take place in the mother's presence unless the baby's condition is poor enough to require special care immediately."
—"Once out, place the baby immediately on the bare skin of my chest. The first examination may take place there after ten minutes of bonding."
—"During the newborn exam, please do not hang our baby upside down or perform any chiropractic maneuvers without consulting us beforehand."

Breastfeeding.

—"My plan is to breastfeed within one hour of birth."
—"If there has been an emergency and the baby is not available to me for breastfeeding, or I am not available to the baby, I would like the assistance of a nurse or aide in expressing my colostrum as soon as possible for the baby."
—"So as not to interfere with early breastfeeding efforts, the baby should be given no artificial milk or water by bottles with artificial nipples, and no pacifiers."

Rooming-in.

—"The baby will stay with me at all times from the moment of birth until we leave the hospital and be placed in a bassinet beside my bed when I cannot hold him."
—"If the baby must be taken from our room for any reason, my husband plans to accompany the baby."

Choose Your Own Language and Format

There is no right way to draft the wording in a birth plan. The suggestions above cover some of the most pressing issues in maternity care—items such as inductions, epidurals, technology, and surgery, but by no means is the list complete. Your plan should be designed for your unique circumstances, so go ahead and phrase your desired features of labor and delivery in your own way. It can be simple, like the following plan.

TITLE: **My Birth Plan**
LOCATION: **Home**
ATTENDANT: **Midwife**
COMPANIONS: **Husband**
MOVEMENT: **Free movement**
LABOR POSITIONS: **Various, making use of gravity**
FOOD AND BEVERAGES: **Yes**
IV: **No**
EPISIOTOMY: **No, I prefer to tear naturally and be sewn up.**
All other procedures should be handled on a case-by-case basis if they arise.
BABY CARE: **Skin-to-skin contact following birth, exam done on mother's chest, breastfeeding**
SICK BABY: **Handled carefully with my full involvement if it arises**

Of course, your plan may include more personal facts and concerns than this one. A short plan, such as this, is really only appropriate for a low-risk home birth, where medications and interventions are under a pregnant woman's control. It is not really detailed enough for a hospital birth. A hospital plan can also be more complicated, like the following plan, which has been slightly modified from a real one.

Birth Plan for Mary and John Smith
To our birth attendants,

We look forward to sharing our first birth experience with you. Preparing ourselves for parenthood has been an intricate experience, and we have absorbed a great deal of information in order to make the wisest decisions. As a direct result of this newfound knowledge, we have established a series of values and priorities that all draw from the same core belief—that we have complete faith in Mary's ability to give birth naturally. We have prepared ourselves for the birth experience we hope for by taking highly informative birth classes and have been practicing the numerous physical and mental techniques involved in the course. Our doula, [NAME OF PRACTITIONER], has been an additional source of information and support.

The concept of informed consent is critical to us. You have already assured us that all decisions are to be discussed and no procedures would be permitted without our approval. John will be the birth advocate, and will be providing physical and emotional support throughout the entire labor and delivery process. If at any time the medical conditions warrant an intervention, we are willing to discuss the proposed intervention as well as the possible alternatives. After discussing the situation, we expect our final decision to be respected and honored, even if it is in opposition to the opinions of others.

Here are some guidelines that describe the birth experience we desire for ourselves and our baby. Please do not deviate from this plan without our consent. We do not expect Mary's labor to be brief or painless, but we do expect her to labor within these specific forms of comfort.

We are relieved and delighted that many of our principles are routine practices families experience while in your care.

Labor and Delivery

- We should not be separated from each other or our doula unless we make the request.

- If an IV is needed, Mary would like it in her arm, not her hand.

- Mary's amniotic membranes should not be artificially ruptured.

- Pelvic exams and fetal monitoring should be kept to a minimum. Monitoring should be done by fetoscope, as it has been proven to be as accurate as electronic monitors and Dopplers.

- Mary would like to labor in a serene atmosphere with dimmed lighting. If speaking is necessary, please communicate in quiet, calm tones.

- Mary will eat light, nonconstipating foods during early labor and clear liquids during labor as well as ice chips and small pieces of frozen honey.

- No drugs of any kind are to be offered to Mary at any point in the process. If a medical necessity requires some form of anesthetic, we will decide at that time what will be used.

- No episiotomy will be performed under any circumstances. Perineal massage with oil, hot compresses, and other forms of perineal support will be employed to prepare her perineal tissues to stretch. In the event that a tear is likely, we prefer the tissues be allowed to tear rather than be cut. Mary would like a local anesthetic if stitches are needed.

- John would like to catch the baby and cut the umbilical cord, if the situation allows it.

- As soon as the baby is delivered, he should be placed skin on skin with Mary and they should not be separated.

Postpartum

- As discussed with head nurse [INSERT NAME OF PRACTITIONER], the three of us should not be separated. All newborn evaluations and care such as bathing and warming should be done in our room.

- We prefer that a nonirritating agent such as erythromycin be used in the baby's eyes after mother and child have had some time to bond. We would like the vitamin K shot given at the same time.

- Our baby should be given no substance by mouth other than Mary's colostrum and breast milk. At no time should sterile water, glucose water, or formula of any kind be given. The baby should be allowed to nurse as she wants to, and no rubber nipples or pacifiers should be given. If the baby's blood sugar level is of concern, more frequent nursing will be encouraged as maternal colostrum provides a more healthy and stable blood sugar level than processed glucose.

- Our baby will not receive a hepatitis B shot while in the hospital. We are planning a vaccination schedule with our pediatrician.

Legal Matters

Your birth plan is a legal document as well as being an agent of communication.

The Evidence-to-Care Gap

Every obstetric textbook instructs that the gold standard of practice today is evidence-based practice. Yet there is a gap between what the scientific evidence shows doctors should be doing and what many are actually doing in hospitals. When obstetricians are asked why, the most frequent answer they give is fear of litigation, a determinant of practice that has nothing to do with a pregnant woman's condition. Unfortunately, this kind of "defensive obstetrics" is widespread. Procedures such as routine electronic fetal monitoring and routine IVs are performed not for a medical indication but as a defense against lawsuits. Surveys have found that the great majority of obstetricians have at one time or another employed such defensive approaches to avoid negligence claims.[1]

In the present legal system, if there is a bad birth outcome, aggrieved clients are permitted to sue their doctors. During the trial, the doctors may then find themselves criticized because they didn't perform interventions such as a cesarean section or EFM. There are relatively few cases of litigation, however, in which doctors find themselves criticized for performing unnecessary interventions. As a result, doctors know they take a risk by *not* doing interventions. They believe they gain insurance against litigation by doing *more* interventions, even those that are not scientifically justified.[2] However, this may be changing.

Recently in Massachusetts, a pregnant woman who'd had a previous cesarean section wanted to have a vaginal birth. During her labor her doctors apparently steered her toward another cesarean through emotional coercion, although she was progressing normally. In court, she claimed they misrepresented the risks of vaginal birth and ignored her pleas to experience it, despite having previously agreed to help her try to achieve a vaginal birth after cesarean. She signed a consent form, but the court upheld that it was not "fully informed" consent that she gave due to the way the doctors spun the risks. The plaintiff won a $1.5 million settlement based on losing her personal decision-making power over her own health and her baby's birth, suffering posttraumatic stress disorder, and loss of consortium with her husband, who was not consulted by doctors on the interpretation of his wife's wishes during childbirth.[3]

There are several problems with defensive obstetrics. First, the fundamental principle of medical practice is that whatever the doctor does must be done foremost for the benefit and interests of the woman. Therefore, if a doctor picks up a scalpel and cuts open a woman's belly, performing a cesarean section because he or she is afraid of going to court or afraid of rising insurance costs, that doctor is not practicing good medicine.

Another problem is that defensive obstetrics treats the symptom (lawsuits), not the disease (damaged patients). Why is there so much litigation? The medical profession often precipitates it by trying out new interventions without waiting to find out if they are safe. All those who practice this unregulated style of obstetrics are simply begging for trouble. Things can, and do, go wrong when doctors don't wait to find out what science proves is safest to do. We've seen this with the use of the ulcer drug Cytotec to kick-start labor. When catastrophes occurred in the past after inductions with Cytotec (such as uterine ruptures, brain-damaged infants, maternal and neonatal mortality), large out-of-court settlements have been made for officially nondisclosed amounts.

Another real cause of litigation is the lack of a satisfactory complaints system for women and families who want information on what went wrong at the birth of their babies and why their requests weren't honored. Having access to such information is called transparency. Transparency and accountability are the new direction in American healthcare services. But attempts to get information from doctors and hospitals are frequently met with stonewalling—and rarely, if ever, with an apology.

There are additional causes of obstetric litigation that you don't hear about from doctors and hospitals. A source of women's dissatisfaction and anger when faced with a birth crisis undoubtedly stems from a broken promise. In order to convince birthing women to give up the comfort and security of their own homes and come to hospitals to give birth, doctors and hospitals have found it necessary to imply through advertising and other means, a perfect birth and a perfect baby.[4] Thus, they're often blamed for the natural disasters as well as for medical mistakes. Nowhere is the mortality rate for women giving birth zero and nowhere is the mortality rate for babies being born zero. Women and babies can get hurt around the time of birth. Throughout history, women have accepted the harsh reality that sometimes accompanies birth, until recently when they began being promised perfect childbirth outcomes.

Protecting Your Interests

When you enter the hospital for childbirth, you will be asked to sign a general consent form. Then, if you are to receive an intervention, such as induction of labor, cesarean section, or epidural anesthesia, you'll be asked to sign additional consent forms. Too often these consent forms do not provide you with "informed consent," as they contain no relevant information. They are presented to you for the purpose of protecting the hospital from litigation. For fully informed consent, which is your legal right, it is important that you be given a written form containing the necessary information on risks and benefits. Remember that by law you can refuse to sign a consent form, or you can modify it (see chapter 3, pages 39–40).

A customized form legally documents your refusal to accept certain treatments and alerts staff that you understand and are prepared to protect your rights. Such a document also requires staff to obtain direct verbal consent from you each time they want to do a procedure that you've already declined in writing. Then you can decide at that time if you believe a particular treatment should or should not be accepted.

The doctrine of informed consent and refusal is upheld by common law, case law, constitutional law, federal law, international tort law, state law and state mandated medical ethics, and the ethical guidelines of the AMA and the ACOG. It provides you with certain fundamental rights,[5] including the right to:

- Exercise self-determination and autonomy in making medical decisions, including the decision to refuse treatment

- Bodily integrity (any form of nonconsensual touching or treatment that occurs in a medical setting constitutes battery)

- Be provided with the necessary information on which to base medical decisions, including a diagnosis; recommended treatments and alternatives; the risks, benefits, discomforts, and potential disabilities of proposed medical treatments; realistic expectation of outcomes; the right to a second opinion, and any financial or research interests a physician may have in proposing certain treatments

- Be informed of any potentially life-threatening consequences of a proposed treatment, even if the likelihood of experiencing such an outcome is rare

- Make medical decisions free from coercion or undue influence from physicians

- Have informed medical decisions witnessed, signed, and documented by the attending physician and another adult

- Revoke consent to treatment at any time, either verbally or in writing

According to the FDA, consent forms for patients participating in an experimental trial of a drug or procedure must adhere to six principles. Making an excellent model for hospital consent forms for the use of *all* drugs and procedures, these principles are as follows:

- Telling you that something is perfectly safe is not appropriate.

- Any reasonably foreseeable risks must be described to you, and the explanations of risk you are given should not minimize reported adverse effects.

- When describing any benefits, consent forms should not contain unproven claims of effectiveness or certainty of benefits, either explicit or implicit, that may unduly influence you. Overly optimistic representations are misleading and violate the requirement to minimize the possibility of coercion. It is common, albeit inappropriate, for consent forms to include only those purposes of the drug or procedure that a patient would consider most beneficial, overstate facts, or are overly favorable in tone or wording.

- The full range of appropriate alternative procedures or courses of treatment that are available must be disclosed. Frequently consent forms fail to adequately describe the treatment alternatives available to the patient or risks and benefits of the alternatives.

- The patient must be told who to contact for answers to pertinent questions.

• The form should include a statement that agreeing to take the drug or use the procedure is voluntary, that refusal will involve no penalty, and that the drug or procedure may be discontinued at any time without penalty.[6]

These six principles are also an important guide for you in asking questions when a hospital staff member suggests a drug or procedure to you. Although it's the duty of any doctor, midwife, or nurse to provide you with full and honest information, you must accept responsibility for asking questions, because you cannot always rely on a maternity-care provider to volunteer such information. Leave no stone unturned. If information does not seem forthcoming and complete, you must demand it. Because your wishes and those of your doctor may collide, it's sometimes difficult to get unbiased information. Another important strategy for eliciting unbiased information is to insist on seeing the scientific data. As I mentioned earlier, "Show me the data" is a powerful request. You are also entitled to a second opinion from a practitioner of your own choosing.

The federal government and a number of states have articulated and protected the right to fully informed consent (or refusal) through various patients' bills of rights.[7] A number of hospitals also have implemented private patient bills of rights that declare their institutional intention to respect patient autonomy and the doctrine of informed consent.

To ensure that your hospital or birthing center adheres to your wishes, consider hiring a midwife to be your primary attendant during labor. There is overwhelming evidence that midwives use far fewer interventions and still have as good, or better, results than obstetricians.[8]

If, for whatever reason, it's not possible for your primary attendant to be a midwife, then it's important to bring someone else along to the hospital who can serve as your advocate. An advocate can be a husband, mother, doula, or friend. This person must be familiar with the elements of your birth plan and your rights. And, hopefully, this person is characteristically confident and unafraid, so that forceful doctors or nurses won't easily sway him or her. With any luck, your advocate won't need to do battle with hospital staff and can simply be present to love and support you for the duration of your birth experience.

A final important strategy for ensuring that your wishes are honored is to document what happens during the birth with a small, handheld video camera. Recording your interactions with hospital staff accomplishes dual purposes. Not only does it send a message that you're serious about your birth plan and intend to hold them responsible in the future for closely adhering to your intentions, it also creates valuable memorabilia for you and your family. If you ask ahead of time and learn that your hospital doesn't permit videotaping of births,[9] you can change hospitals, raise your insistence with the hospital administration, or contact the local media.

What to Do If You Have a Complaint Before or During Labor

If you plan to give birth in a specific hospital and discover ahead of time that the staff is unwilling to comply with your wishes, as might conceivably happen if, let's say, you were planning to give birth vaginally after a cesarean section, you are entitled to file a complaint with the hospital's chief compliance officer. If the hospital has no one serving in a position with that exact job title, telephone the hospital switchboard and ask to receive the information necessary to file a complaint as well as the name of a contact.

According to Katherine Prown, Ph.D., advocacy director of ICAN, hospitals that receive federal funding (approximately 80 percent of them) must adhere to the Center for Medicare and Medicaid Service's (CMS) conditions of participation (CoP). These require hospitals to honor patient rights for *all* patients as these rights are defined by the Patient Self-Determination Act, the Consumer Bill of Rights and Responsibilities, EMTALA, and a large body of case law upholding the right to refuse treatment, to be fully informed of the risks, benefits, and alternatives of any proposed treatment, and to participate in all treatment decisions.

Hospitals that fail to adhere are subject to heavy fines and risk losing their right to qualify for Medicare and Medicaid funding. The CoP also require that hospitals institute an internal grievance process and give patients the information they need to know about how to file a complaint and where to appeal in the case of an unfavorable ruling.[10]

Under the CoP, a hospital must respond to your initial complaint within one week or else offer you an explanation of the reasons for the delay and provide an estimated time frame for a response. Failure to do so is in itself a violation. If the hospital's chief compliance officer or another designated person issues an unfavorable ruling, then your next step is to appeal to the Office of the Inspector General at the Department of Health and Human Services (HHS). If HHS also rules in favor of the hospital, then you can make an appeal to the Department of Justice. Many patients have had success using this complaints procedure. For example, deaf patients denied interpreters by hospitals in violation of the CoP have successfully used this grievance process to hold hospitals accountable for violating their rights as patients under federal law.

As a maternity services consumer, it is important to know the best procedures to follow to get your needs met before you need them (and hopefully you won't). When you visit the hospital before giving birth, ask your tour guide some questions so that you and your birth advocate will come to the hospital prepared to negotiate your care. Try asking simple, straightforward questions like:

- "If I find I need something during childbirth, with whom should I speak?"

- "If I have questions during birth whom should I ask?"

- "Whose job is it to handle patient affairs and complaints?"

- "Is there a patient liaison whose duties include addressing patient questions?"

It is also important to determine during your pregnancy if the hospital you have chosen must adhere to the CoP.

Once you're in labor, it's typical that the main person with whom you'll need to negotiate elements of your care is a labor-and-delivery nurse. If you and the nurses assigned to your care cannot reach an agreement, you or a birth advocate will have to go up the "chain of command" to get satisfaction. What should you do, for instance, if you and your partner want to videotape your baby's birth and the nurses won't allow it? Or if you do not want an IV and the staff is insisting? First, ask to speak with the nursing supervisor. Then, ask to speak with your attending physician. If you still don't reach an agreement about your care, contact the hospital administration. If you "go up the chain" and your problem is not resolved, then ask to be introduced into the complaints system.

Can you force doctors, nurses, and hospitals to comply with your wishes for labor and delivery? If your complaints made during pregnancy have not been successfully resolved, there is another strategy available to you at the time of giving birth. You can invoke your legal rights under EMTALA and the CoP. Originally enacted in 1986 to prevent "patient dumping" (such as refusing to admit a woman in labor for any reason, including lack of ability to pay for services), under the EMTALA patients requiring emergency care cannot be transferred to another hospital until after they are "stabilized." In the case of women in labor, this is defined as the delivery of both baby and placenta.[11]

EMTALA applies once you set foot within 250 feet of the hospital. The hospital must admit you. Then, if you're admitted to the hospital and the nurses or physicians fail to inform you of the risks, benefits, and alternatives to a proposed intervention, the CoP protect your interests.

Any woman who finds herself laboring in an adversarial situation or confronting non-compliance with her wishes should repeatedly use such phrases as "It's my right under the conditions of participation to decline a, b, or c procedures" or "If you perform an intervention without my consent, I plan to file a complaint for violating my legal rights under CoP."[12] If staff members you are dealing with respond, "What is CoP?" you may need to educate them. Your next statement should be, "I need to speak to someone in the administration who knows about the Center for Medicare and Medicaid Service's Emergency Medical Treatment and Active Labor Act and the Center's conditions of participation, the regulations that protect my rights as a patient." This is a mouthful, of course, which is why it is important for you to have an advocate.

Remember, invoking EMTALA and the CoP is a last-ditch strategy. As a consumer, you need to know your rights and what to do if they are being violated. But I hope you never need to apply this information and find an easier, less stressful way to get your needs met.

Is Your Birth Plan a Binding Legal Document?

If you present your birth plan to a hospital staff and they don't follow it, what are your grounds for a legal complaint? Here are a few legal scenarios you might encounter:

1• *They do not tell you that they aren't following the plan.* The issue is informed consent. You have grounds for complaint if there is an adverse outcome.

2• *They don't follow the plan, but they* do *inform you ahead of time that they are deviating from it.* The issue, again, is informed consent. You would only have grounds for a complaint if there were an adverse outcome and you can prove you were not fully informed of the risks and benefits of the procedures they used.

3• *The hospital staff does a procedure without your consent.* The issue is civil battery. No one is allowed to do a medical procedure on you without your informed consent. Nonetheless, you have no grounds for a lawsuit unless there is an adverse outcome.

In a life-threatening emergency, under the law, the consent issue holds no water. Professional caregivers are required to act, using their full skills and abilities, and best judgment, to counter the threat at hand. That protects you from harm, as well as them. Courts can only order so-called damages to be paid when there is an adverse physical outcome. Emotional reasons are not usually considered worthy of remuneration, although posttraumatic stress syndrome after birth has been worthy of remuneration on occasion. But there is recourse available to seriously dissatisfied and unhappy parents who feel they were neglected or violated in some manner, or whose wishes were ignored or maliciously overridden. If a staff person has seen your birth plan and it is not followed, and there are no adverse outcomes, you can sue that individual and/or facility for breach of contract. But you could only ever get professional fees back on these grounds, never damages. Such cases are usually litigated in small claims court.

My opinion is that women who want the safest, most empowering births should choose to labor at home or in an out-of-hospital setting under the care of a midwife. The midwives' model of care rarely becomes confrontational or as disappointing as medical care at its worst is prone to become, as the former starts from the assumption that pregnancy and birth are a normal part of life rather than a disease. If you choose a midwife as a birth attendant, you know she is committed to the following principles (articulated by the Midwifery Task Force), which are proven to reduce the incidence of birth injury, trauma, and surgery.[13]

- Monitoring your physical, psychological, and social well-being

- Providing you with individualized education, counseling, and prenatal care, continuous hands-on assistance during labor and delivery, and postpartum support

- Minimizing technological interventions

- Identifying and referring you to a doctor if you require obstetrical attention[14]

Ultimately, it is up to you to decide what you do and do not want to include in your birth plan, and what measures you feel would ensure your safety and satisfaction. You have many choices of caregivers and birthplaces. You've been told about the legal matters surrounding your birth plan because, as an informed consumer, you need to know that overly medical childbirth and childbirth that ignores women's preferences exists. You need to be prepared so you can either avoid it or stand up to it. But frankly, I am suggesting that you prepare for an occurrence that hopefully you will not encounter.

On a Final, More Uplifting Note

Without question, childbirth is going to be one of the major events in your life. I want it to be an uplifting and transformative experience, a memory worth treasuring. Now that you are fully informed about what can happen during childbirth, let me also assure you that you can, perhaps with some effort, find a woman-centered and mother-friendly environment in which to have a joyous birth experience.

Many wonderful midwives and obstetricians exist who truly want to support you in the awesome and life-changing process of having a baby, and they would be delighted for you to share your most intimate wishes and birth plan with them. So please, take your birth plan in hand, go and find those great and helpful practitioners, and may you then take pleasure in the safe, joyous, fulfilling, and empowering childbirth of your dreams.

Resources

Midwives Alliance of North America
(MANA)
375 Rockbridge Road, Suite 172-313
Lilburn, GA 30047
(888) 923-MANA (toll-free)
Email: info@mana.org
www.mana.org

American College of Nurse-Midwives
(ACNM)
8403 Colesville Road, Suite 1550
Silver Spring, MD 20910
(240) 485-1800
Email: info@acnm.org
www.midwife.org

North American Registry of
Midwives
5257 Rosestone Drive
Lilburn, GA 30047
(888) 842-4784 (toll-free)
www.narm.org

DONA International
P.O. Box 626
Jasper, IN 47547
(888) 788-DONA (toll-free)
www.dona.org

Association of Labor Assistants and
Childbirth Educators
P.O. Box 382724
Cambridge, MA 02238-2724

(888) 222-5223 (toll-free)
www.alace.org

International Childbirth Education
Association (ICEA)
P.O. Box 20048
Minneapolis, MN 55420
(952) 854-8660
www.icea.org

Birth Policy (includes state-by-state
resources)
www.birthpolicy.org

Childbirth Connection (formerly
Maternity Center Association)
281 Park Avenue South
New York, NY 10010
(212) 777-5000
Email: info@maternitywise.org
www.maternitywise.org

U.S. Centers for Disease Control and
Prevention/National Center for Health
Statistics
1600 Clifton Road
Atlanta, GA 30333
(800) 311-3435 (toll-free)
www.cdc.gov

National Institutes of Health
9000 Rockville Pike
Bethesda, MD 20892

(301) 496-4000
www.nih.gov

National Association of Childbearing Centers (NACC)
3123 Gottschall Road
Perkiomenville, PA 18074-9546
(215) 234-8068
www.birthcenters.org

Midwifery Today
P.O. Box 2672
Eugene, OR 97402
(800) 743-0974 (toll-free)
www.midwiferytoday.com

National Association of Postpartum Care Services
800 Detroit Street
Denver, CO 80206
(800) 45-DOULA (toll-free)
www.napcs.org

International Cesarean Awareness Network (ICAN)
1304 Kingsdale Avenue
Redondo Beach, CA 90278
(310) 542-6400
(800) 686-ICAN (toll-free)
www.ican-online.org

International Lactation Consultant Association
1500 Sunday Drive, Suite 102
Raleigh, NC 27607
(919) 861-5577
www.ilca.org

La Leche League
1400 North Meacham Road
Schaumburg, IL 60173-4048
(847) 519-7730
(800) LA-LECHE (toll-free)
www.lalecheleague.org

Coalition for Improving Maternity Services (CIMS)
P.O. Box 2346

Ponte Vedra Beach, FL 32004
(888) 282-CIMS (toll-free)
www.motherfriendly.org

Association of Nurse Advocates for Childbirth Solutions (ANACS)
916 Daleview Drive
Silver Spring, MD 20901
(301) 434-5546
www.anacs.org

Association of Women's Health, Obstetric and Neonatal Nurses (AWHONN)
2000 L Street, NW, Suite 740
Washington, DC 20036
(202) 261-2400
(800) 673-8499 (toll-free)
www.awhonn.org

Citizens for Midwifery (CFM)
P.O. Box 82227
Athens, GA 30608-2227
(888) CFM-4880
www.cfmidwifery.org

American Public Health Association (APHA)
800 I Street, NW
Washington, DC 20001-3710
(202) 777-APHA
www.apha.org

U.S. Cochrane Center/The Cochrane Collaboration
169 Angell Street
Box G-S2
Providence, RI 02912
(401) 863-9950
www.cochrane.us
www.cochrane.org
www.thecochranelibrary.com

Lamaze International
2025 M Street, Suite 800
Washington, DC 20036
(800) 368-4404
www.lamaze.org

Notes

Introduction

1. Despite our faith in technology and doctors, statistics show that fifteen countries have lower maternal mortality rates than does the United States. In order: Sweden, Japan, Ireland, New Zealand, Slovakia, Portugal, Austria, Italy, Spain, Finland, Canada, Germany, Yugoslavia, Greece, and Denmark (source: World Health Organization). Twenty-one countries have lower newborn mortality rates than we do.

Chapter 1

1. The Coalition for Improving Maternity Services (CIMS) is a group of individuals and organizations sharing concern for the care and well-being of mothers, babies, and families. CIMS, a United Nations–recognized nongovernmental organization, was formed in 1996 and has more than fifty organizational members, including groups of midwives, labor-and-delivery nurses, doulas, childbirth educators, and others, all together representing more than 90,000 individuals. Their mission is to promote a wellness model of maternity care that will improve birth outcomes and substantially reduce costs. "Ten Steps of the Mother-Friendly Childbirth Initiative for Mother-Friendly Hospitals, Birth Centers, and Home Birth Services," copyright © 1996 by the Coalition for Improving Maternity Services (CIMS). Website: www.motherfriendly.org.

2. According to the Ten Steps of the Mother-Friendly Childbirth Initiative, hospitals, birth centers, and home-birth services should not exceed the following rates of interventions: an induction rate of 10 percent or less; an episiotomy rate of 20 percent or less, with a goal of 5 percent or less; a total cesarean rate of 10 percent or less in community hospitals and 15 percent or less in tertiary care (high-risk) hospitals; and a VBAC rate of 60 percent or more with a goal of 75 percent or more.

3. E. Hemminki, "A Trial of Continuous Human Support During Labor: Feasibility, Interventions and Mother's Satisfaction," *Journal of Psychosomatic Obstetrics and Gynecology*, 11(1990): 239–50.

Chapter 2

1. Hemminki, 239–50.
2. "Fetal Heart Rate Patterns: Monitoring, Interpretation and Management," *ACOG Technical Bulletin Number 207*, July 1995.
3. M. Enkin et al., *A Guide to Effective Care in Pregnancy and Childbirth* (New York: Oxford University Press, 2000), 292–94, 503.
4. M. Klaus, *Maternal–Infant Bonding* (St Louis: Mosby, 1976).
5. Enkin et al., 317.
6. Enkin et al., 259–63, 503.

Chapter 3

1. The U.S. Centers for Disease Control and Prevention, National Center for Health Statistics. Website: www.cdc.gov/nchs.
2. K. Prown, "Forcing doctors and hospitals to comply during labor and delivery." Website: www.birthpolicy.org.
3. Any remaining doubts about the safety of home birth were conclusively erased by the publication of a very large, scientifically valid study of more than 5,000 planned home births with midwives: K. Johnson and B. Daviss, "Outcomes of Planned Home Births with Certified Professional Midwives: Large Prospective Study in North America," *British Medical Journal* 330 (June 2005): 1416.
4. Critics of home birth often skew the evidence about the safety of home birth by rolling together statistics on planned home births and unplanned home births.
5. Johnson and Daviss, 1416.

Chapter 4

1. CDC/NCHS. Website: www.cdc.gov/nchs.
2. Henci Goer, *The Thinking Woman's Guide to a Better Birth* (New York: Perigee, 1999), 179.
3. Even the American College of Obstetricians and Gynecologists recommends using the stethoscope on low-risk women because of the high rate of false positive results with the electronic fetal monitor. "Fetal Heart Rate Patterns: Monitoring, Interpretation and Management." *ACOG Technical Bulletin Number 207*, July 1995.
4. M. Wagner, "Fish Can't See Water: The Need to Humanize Birth," *International Journal of Gynecology and Obstetrics* 75 (November 2001), S1: 25–37.
5. M. MacDorman and G. Singh, "Midwifery Care, Social and Medical Risk Factors, and Birth Outcomes in the USA," *Journal of Epidemiology and Community Health* 52 (May 1998): 310–17.

Chapter 5

1. When I give lectures on childbirth, I usually show a projection of the following table that illustrates how often the maternity care in American hospitals deviates from the practices that scientific evidence has proven to be warranted—meaning the evidence-based practices decrease the risk of complications to mother and baby. Percentages based on actual practices are drawn from "Listening to Mothers," the first national survey of childbearing women in the United States, which was published in 2002 by the Maternity Center Association (now known as Childbirth Connection). Percentages based on the best scientific evidence are drawn from Murray Enkin et al., *A Guide to Effective Care in Pregnancy and Childbirth* and the Cochrane Library website: www.cochranelibrary.com.

As this table makes plain, women often don't receive evidence-based treatment, which indicates that they're being made uncomfortable during childbirth for no good reason—and in some instances they and their babies are being placed at higher risk. In addition, the fees charged for experiencing high-tech birth scenarios are higher.

Is Obstetric Care Provided in U.S. Hospitals Evidence Based?

PROCEDURE	ACTUAL PRACTICE	SCIENTIFIC PRACTICE
One continuous labor attendant	< 10%	100%
Routine midwife care	9%	80%
Routine EFM	93%	No
Withholding food or drink	86%	No
Routine IV	86%	No
Confined to bed during all or part of labor	69%	No
Lithotomy (on back with feet in stirrups, near the end of labor)	Nearly all	No
Vacuum or forceps	13%	< 10%
Episiotomy	35%	< 20%
Induce labor with drugs	44%	< 10%
Accelerate ongoing labor with drugs	53%	< 10%
Cesarean section	29.2%	10–15%

2. Enkin et al., 285.
3. Ibid.
4. "Fetal Heart Rate Patterns: Monitoring, Interpretation and Management."
5. Enkin et al., chapter 30.
6. From "Listening to Mothers" (Maternity Center Association survey).
7. Ibid.

Chapter 6
1. CDC/NCHS. Website: www.cdc.gov/nchs.
2. When is a postterm baby in jeopardy? A study published in 1963 found that the number of babies dying inside the uterus increased slightly at forty-two weeks and significantly after forty-three weeks (J. McClure-Brown, "Postmaturity," *American Journal of Obstetrics and Gynecology* 85 (1963): 373). That study began the move in obstetrics to induce labor if a pregnancy has gone more than forty-two weeks. Yet only 3 percent of women go beyond forty-two weeks. Induction reveals a characteristic of obstetric practice: the bandwagon effect. Everyone jumps on the wagon, which goes faster and faster, and then they're afraid to get off.

Later, good research studies done in 1982 and in 1987 found no significant increase in fetal mortality after forty-two weeks, and only a slight increase even after forty-three weeks (R. L. Williams et al., "Fetal Growth and Perinatal Viability in California," *Obstetrics and Gynecology* 59 (1982): 624. Also: R. D. Eden et al., "Perinatal Characteristics in Uncomplicated Postdated Pregnancies," *Obstetrics and Gynecology* 69 (1987): 306. Another valid study published in 1996 of almost 1,800 post-term pregnancies found no increase in fetal deaths and no increase in complications of birth when the pregnancies were compared to babies born "on time" between thirty-seven and forty-one weeks (D. Weinstein et al., "Expectant Management of Post-Term Patients: Observations and Outcome," *Journal of Maternal Fetal Medicine* 5(5) (1996): 293–97.

Obstetricians communicate fear to pregnant women when telling them, both directly and indirectly, by performing numerous tests, all that might go wrong: The baby might suddenly die in the uterus, the baby's heart might suddenly stop, and so forth. Of course, legal consent forms must list every disaster that could potentially happen. When induction is suggested, the idea is appealing to a woman because it means that the supposedly dangerous situation for her baby—remaining inside her womb—might end sooner. At that moment, she is not necessarily being told the unvarnished truth that carrying her baby for as long as possible makes it stronger.

For an excellent review of the indications for induction and the evolution of labor induction, see "Induction and Circular Logic," by Gail Hart, *Midwifery Today* 63 (Autumn 2002): 24.

3. Macrosomia is not listed as an indication for induction of labor by the American College of Obstetricians and Gynecologists. "Induction of Labor," *ACOG Practice Bulletin Number 10*, November 1999.

4. Enkin et al., 75–78.

5. Enkin et al., chapter 32.

6. L. L. Albers, M. Schiff, and J. G. Gorwoda, "The Length of Active Labor in Normal Pregnancies," *Obstetrics and Gynecology* 87(3) (1996): 355–59. Also see Goer, chapter 7.

7. In human physiology, a minute difference in a molecule can make a huge difference in effect. Prostaglandin 1 and prostaglandin 2 have a slight difference in their molecules and they produce different effects. Unlike Cytotec (prostaglandin 1, or the generic misoprostol), prostaglandin 2 drugs have been through the correct FDA evaluation process to determine safety.

8. M. Wagner, *Pursuing the Birth Machine* (Camperdown, Australia: ACE Graphics, 1994), 136.

9. The increased risk of uterine rupture with using uterine stimulant drugs for labor induction is well established and a warning of the risk of uterine rupture appears with the package insert that comes with the drugs, and both the FDA and the pharmaceutical company have issued warnings of this risk. The risk of amniotic fluid embolism when using uterine stimulant drugs for induction of labor has been confirmed by a careful scientific review of the evidence. M. Wagner, "From Caution to Certainty: Hazards in the Formation of Evidence-Based Practice," *Pediatric and Perinatal Epidemiology* 19(2) (2005): 173–76.

10. The Cochrane Library, 1995 through 2004. Website: www.cochranelibrary.com.

11. M. Wagner, "Adverse Events Following Misoprostol Induction of Labor." *Midwifery Today* 71 (2004): 9–12.

Chapter 7

1. Enkin et al. 328.

2. Ina May Gaskin, *Ina May's Guide to Childbirth*, 150–53.

3. Enkin et al., 315.

4. Goer, 126.

5. There are three excellent studies on the risks associated with epidurals: B. Leighton and S. Halpern. "The Effects of Epidural Anesthesia on Labor, Maternal and Neonatal Outcomes," *American Journal of Obstetrics and Gynecology* 186 (2002): 569–77; E. Lieberman, and C. O'Donoghue, "Unintended Effects of Epidural Anesthesia During Labor," *American Journal of Obstetrics and Gynecology* 186 (2002): 531–68; and L. Mayberry and D. Clemmens, "Epidural Analgesia Side Effects, Co-Interventions, and Care of Women During Childbirth," *American Journal of Obstetrics and Gynecology* 186 (2002): 581–93.

6. Enkin et al., 324.

7. Enkin et al., chapter 34; and Goer, chapter 8.

8. Ibid.

9. Ibid.

10. *Ob. Gyn. News*, as cited by Goer, 129.

Chapter 8

1. J. A. Martin, B. E. Hamilton, F. Menacker, P. D. Sutton, and T. J. Mathews, "Preliminary Births for 2004: Infant and Maternal Health," Health E-stats, November 15, 2005. See the U.S. Centers for Disease Control and Prevention/National Center for Health Statistics. Website: www.cdc.gov/nchs.

2. For a discussion of the process by which the World Health Organization determined the optimal cesarean section rate in 1985, see M. Wagner, "Fish Can't See Water: The Need to Humanize Birth," *International Journal of Gynecology and Obstetrics* 75 (2001): supplements 25–37. For more recent confirmation see A. P. Betrán, M. Merialdi, J. A. Lauer, W. Bing-shun, J. Thomas, P. Van Look, and M. Wagner, "Rates of Caesarean Section: Analysis of Global, Regional and National Estimates." Presented at the Second International Conference on Humanization of Birth, Rio de Janiero, Brazil, November 2005. Submitted for publication.

3. Goer, 55.

4. The scientific literature on the risks of urinary and fecal incontinence after vaginal birth is reviewed in the paper: M. Wagner, "Critique of British Royal College of Obstetricians and Gynaecologists National Sentinel Caesarean Section Audit Report of October 2001," *MIDIRS Journal*, September 2002.

5. An excellent, scientifically sound, and thorough discussion of vaginal birth after cesarean (VBAC) and why it is a safe option is found on the International Cesarean Awareness Network website: www.ican-online.org.

6. M. Wagner, "Choosing Caesarean Section," *The Lancet* 356 (2000): 1677–80.

7. Ibid.

8. By far the most reliable source of information on the risks of women dying from emergency cesarean section and elective cesarean section is Marion H. Hall and Susan Bewley, "Maternal Mortality and Mode of Delivery," *The Lancet* 354 (1999): 776. (This paper used data from the British confidential enquiries on maternal mortality.)

9. Ibid.

10. Wagner, "Choosing Caesarean Section."

11. Ibid.

12. J. A. Martin et al.

13. For a discussion of the many risks of cesarean section to women and to babies, documented with references to the scientific literature, see Wagner "Choosing Caesarean Section."

14. M. Wagner, "Midwifery in the Industrialized World," *Journal of the Society of Obstetricians and Gynecologists of Canada* 20(13) (1998): 1225–34.
15. Enkin et al., 190.
16. S. Chauhan, H. Roach, et al., "Cesarean Section for Suspected Fetal Distress: Does the Decision-Incision Time Make a Difference?" *Journal of Reproductive Medicine* 42(6) (1997): 347–52.
17. "Listening to Mothers."
18. Enkin et al., 293.
19. K. Hartmann et al., "Outcome of Routine Episiotomy: A Systematic Review," *Journal of the American Medical Association* 293 (2005): 2141–48.
20. Ibid.
21. Ibid.
22. Ibid.
23. See Wagner, "Critique of British Royal College of Obstetricians and Gynaecologists National Sentinel Caesarean Section Audit Report of October 2001."
24. Hartmann et al.

Chapter 9
1. Wagner, *Pursuing the Birth Machine,* 96–100.
2. The U.S. Centers for Disease Control and Prevention, National Center for Health Statistics. Website: www.cdc.gov/nchs.
3. Enkin et al., 146.
4. Ibid.
5. Enkin et al., 188.
6. M. Hannah, "Planned Cesarean Section versus Planned Vaginal Birth in Singleton Breech Birth," *The Lancet* 356 (2000): 1375–83.
7. M. Glezeman, "Five Years to the Term Breech Trial: The Rise and Fall of a Randomized Controlled Trial," *American Journal of Obstetrics and Gynecology* 194 (1) (2006): 20–25.
8. Enkin et al., 173.
9. Enkin et al., 75–77.
10. Ibid.
11. The U.S. Centers for Disease Control and Prevention, National Center for Health Statistics. Website: www.cdc.gov/nchs.
12. M. Cedergren, "Maternal Morbid Obesity and the Risk of Adverse Outcomes," *Obstetrics and Gynecology* 103 (2004): 219–24.
13. Ibid.
14. The U.S. Centers for Disease Control and Prevention, National Center for Health Statistics. Website: www.cdc.gov/nchs.
15. National Institute of Child Health and Development. Website: www.nichd.nih.gov.
16. The U.S. Centers for Disease Control and Prevention, National Center for Health Statistics. Website: www.cdc.gov/nchs.
17. A number of good articles on the emotional impact of childhood sexual abuse and rape on women during the experience of labor are available online from the archives of Gentle Birth. See: R. Spindler, "Childhood Sexual Abuse and Its Effects on Childbirth." Website: www.gentlebirth.org/archives/abusepaper.html.

Chapter 10

1. E. D. Hodnett, S. Gates, G. J. Hofmeyr, and C. Sakala, "Continuous Support for Women During Childbirth (Review)," *The Cochrane Library* (2005), 1. See Childbirth Connection website: www.childbirthconnection.org.
2. Enkin et al., 253.
3. Enkin et al., 249.
4. Penny Simkin, founder of DONA International, quoted in *Pregnancy Today* by Jillian Hanson.
5. Statistics provided by Heidi Rinehart, M.D., in an interview on April 21, 2004.
6. In more than twenty-five years as a specialist in maternity care I have neither met nor heard of a male doula in any country I have visited.
7. See the Seattle Midwifery School website: www.seattlemidwifery.org.
8. For information on doulas, including scientific evidence on the benefits they provide, visit the DONA International website: www.dona.org.

Chapter 11

1. Wagner, *Pursuing the Birth Machine*, 261–63.
2. Wagner, *Pursuing the Birth Machine*, 218, citing T. Field S. Schanberg, F. Scafidi, et al., "Tactile/Kinesthetic Stimulation Effects on Preterm Neonates," *Pediatrics* 77(5) (1986): 654–58.
3. Wagner, *Pursuing the Birth Machine*, 217, citing U. Hunziker and R. Barr, "Increased Carrying Reduces Infant Crying: A Randomized Controlled Trial," *Pediatrics* 77(5) (1986): 641–48.
4. Wagner, *Pursuing the Birth Machine*, 249.
5. Wagner, *Pursuing the Birth Machine*, 261–63.
6. Wagner, *Pursuing the Birth Machine*, 241.
7. Baby-Friendly USA. Website: www.babyfriendlyusa.org.
8. Ibid.
9. For more information on "The Ten Steps to Successful Breastfeeding for Hospitals" as outlined by WHO/UNICEF, and to receive a listing of baby-friendly hospitals in the United States, visit the website of Baby-Friendly USA: www.babyfriendlyusa.org.

Chapter 12

1. Enkin et al., 466.
2. Three studies cited in chapter 6 apply here as well: Leighton and Halpern, 569–77; Lieberman and O'Donoghue, 531–68; and Mayberry and Clemmens, 581–93.
3. Goer, 125–48.
4. Ibid.
5. A. D'Oliveria, "Violence Against Women in Health-Care Institutions: An Emerging Problem," *The Lancet* 359 (May 11, 2002): 1681–85. The authors analyzed rigorous research from the past decade and found four forms of violent abuse of women by doctors and nurses: neglect, verbal abuse, physical abuse, and sexual abuse. They note: "These forms of violence recur, are often deliberate, are a serious violation of human rights, and are related to poor quality and effectiveness of health-care services. This abuse is a means of controlling patients that is learned during training and reinforced in health facilities. Abuse occurs mainly in situations in which the legitimacy of health services is questionable or can be the result of prejudice against certain population groups." The authors

also discuss ways to prevent violent abuse. This paper is an important contribution to our understanding of hospital maternity services and should be read by every obstetrician, midwife, and obstetric nurse.

6. Wagner, *Pursuing the Birth Machine*, 251. Also P. Romito, "Unhappiness After Childbirth," from *A Guide to Effective Care in Pregnancy and Childbirth*, 436–438.

7. Goer, 24–25.

8. M. Garel, "Psychological Consequences of Cesarean Childbirth in Primiparas," *Journal of Psychosomatic Obstetrics and Gynecology* 6 (1987): 197–209. Also Goer, 180.

Chapter 13

1. Physicians openly admit that fear of litigation plays a role in the decision that some hospitals and doctors make not to provide women with the option of vaginal birth after cesarean. An administrator from Frederick Memorial Hospital in Maryland is quoted in an article: R. Stein, "Once a C-Section, Always a C-Section? Women Who Want to Try Labor on Later Deliveries Are Increasingly Refused," *The Washington Post*, November 24, 2005, A24. "'Patient safety is the most important factor,' said Edwin Chen, who heads the obstetrics department. 'But we also had to be concerned about the danger of being sued and going bankrupt. Then we couldn't provide any care to anyone.'" Also *ICAN e-News*, November 23, 2005, 32.

2. Here are two examples of increases in practices driven by fear of litigation rather than scientific evidence. On using cesarean section for breech births: "Physicians in the U.S., facing increased medical-legal pressures, performed fewer vaginal breech deliveries" (and therefore more cesarean section for breech), from *ACOG Practice Bulletin Number 5*, July 1999, 1. On doing repeat cesarean sections rather than assisting women with vaginal birth after cesarean: "Increasingly, these adverse events during trial of labor have lead to malpractice suits. These developments have led to a more circumspect approach to trial of labor," also from *ACOG Practice Bulletin Number 5*, 2. This same *ACOG Bulletin* indicates that the evidence shows 60 to 80 percent of pregnant women can have a successful trial of labor after previous cesarean and yet, according to the CDC, only 9.2 percent had VBAC in 2004, which is a decrease from 67 percent in 1996.

3. From an article by Harold J. Bursztjan, M.D., a member of the Harvard Medical School faculty, posted on the website: www.forensic-psych.com.

4. The statements "childbirth has become very safe" and "couples' expectation of a perfect baby" both come from the same article: B. Sachs et al., "The Risks of Lowering the Cesarean-Delivery Rate," *New England Journal of Medicine* 340(1) (1999): 54–57.

5. K. Prown, "Childbirth and the Law." Website: www.birthpolicy.org.

6. The U.S. Food and Drug Administration has issued guidelines defining informed consent for the protection of human subjects in clinical experiments that also apply to informed consent in medical practice. Regulations are available online: www.fda.gov.

7. The Patient Self-Determination Act (www.dgcenter.org/acp/pdf/psda.pdf) mandates that hospitals must inform patients of their rights upon admission, and in states, such as New York and others, federally protected patient rights are expanded on an reiterated through a statewide patients' bill of rights that includes detailed stipulations regarding maternity care and outlines the various grievance procedures available to women whose hospitals fail to provide the care outlined in the statute. New York State Department of Health website: www.health.state.ny.us/nysdoh/consumer/patient/patient.htm.

8. Wagner, "Midwifery in the Industrialized World," 1225–34.

9. On the subject of parents videotaping their children's births, the article "Liability Implications of Recording Procedures or Treatments," *ACOG Committee Opinion Number 207*, September 1998, states: "Recording solely for the purposes of patient memorabilia or marketing is not without liability, and each institution should weigh these competing concerns. The Committee on Professional Liability strongly discourages any recording of medical or surgical procedures for patient memorabilia."

10. For a summary of patients' rights under the Center for Medicare and Medicaid Service's conditions of participation (CoP) and how they're protected (this protects *all* patients) go to the U.S. Department of Health and Human Services website: www.hhs.gov/news/press/1999pres/990412.html.

   The CoP regulations, including procedures for filing grievances, are available through the U.S. Government Printing Office website, on the Code of Federal Regulation's main website: www.gpoaccess.gov/cfr/index.html.

11. EMTALA is a particularly effective tool for pregnant women who have no other options (for instance, there is no other hospital in their community, or they are in the armed services, or they are a member of a managed care organization that will not comply with their wishes) or who have exhausted other options (such as going to another hospital), and therefore plan to go in labor to the hospital which has stated it will not comply with their wishes for labor and delivery.

12. The Center for Medicare and Medicaid Service is in charge of enforcing EMTALA. To find out where to report a violation in your state, go to: www.medlaw.com/healthlaw/EMTALA/reporting/where-to-report-violation.shtml.

   To read the EMTALA statute and regulations, and get more information, go to: www.medlaw.com/healthlaw/EMTALA/index.shtml.

13. The Midwives Model of Care, copyright © 1996–2004, Midwifery Task Force, Inc., is a definition of midwife care created so that groups of midwives could communicate better with healthcare decision-makers. According to a history on the Citizens for Midwifery website (www.cfmidwifery.org), the group started with the assumption that decision-makers were mainstream and did not think in terms of women being capable decision-makers, and they aimed to address concerns about safety.

14. Ibid.

Index